Ampakine schiz 88
Acamprosate addic 117
Rolipram dep 172
BDNF-MAPK inhib dep 173
Xanomeline SDAT 219
Memantine SDAT 220

Brain Circuitry and Signaling in Psychiatry

Basic Science and Clinical Implications

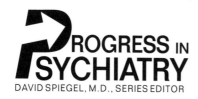

PROGRESS IN PSYCHIATRY

DAVID SPIEGEL, M.D., SERIES EDITOR

Number 61

Brain Circuitry and Signaling in Psychiatry

Basic Science and Clinical Implications

Edited by

Gary B. Kaplan, M.D.
Ronald P. Hammer Jr., Ph.D.

2002

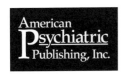

American Psychiatric Publishing, Inc.

Washington, DC
London, England

Note: The authors have worked to ensure that all information in this book concerning drug dosages, schedules, and routes of administration is accurate as of the time of publication and consistent with standards set by the U.S. Food and Drug Administration and the general medical community. As medical research and practice advance, however, therapeutic standards may change. For this reason and because human and mechanical errors sometimes occur, we recommend that readers follow the advice of a physician who is directly involved in their care or the care of a member of their family. A product's current package insert should be consulted for full prescribing and safety information.

Books published by American Psychiatric Publishing, Inc., represent the views and opinions of the individual authors and do not necessarily represent the policies and opinions of APPI or the American Psychiatric Association.

Manufactured in the United States of America on acid-free paper
06 05 04 03 02   5 4 3 2 1
First Edition

American Psychiatric Publishing, Inc.
1400 K Street, N.W.
Washington, DC 20005
www.appi.org

Library of Congress Cataloging-in-Publication Data
Brain circuitry and signaling in psychiatry : basic science and clinical implications / edited by Gary B. Kaplan, Ronald P. Hammer Jr.
    p. cm.
    Includes bibliographical references and index.
    ISBN 0-88048-957-X (alk. paper)
    1. Biological psychiatry. 2. Neural circuitry. 3. Mental illness—Pathophysiology. I. Kaplan, Gary B., 1957–   II. Hammer, Ronald P.
    [DNLM: 1. Biological Psychiatry—methods. 2. Mental Disorders—physiopathology. 3. Brain—physiology. 4. Neural Pathways.
    5. Psychotropic Drugs—therapeutic use. 6. Synaptic Transmission.
    WM 102 N494 2002]
    RC343 .N425 2002
    616.89'07—dc21   2001041365

British Library Cataloguing in Publication Data
A CIP record is available from the British Library.

For Kim, Eliza, and Julia, with love—GK

To my mentors in neuroscience and psychiatric research,
   Marian Diamond and Arnold Scheibel
As always, my gratitude to Sandra Jacobson for her inspiration—RH

Contents

7

9

11 *Neural Circuitry + Signaling
in Attentional D/O*

Contributors

Ari Blitz, M.D.
Fellow, Howard Hughes Medical Institute–National Institutes of Health Research Scholars Program and Program in Liberal Medical Education, Brown Medical School, Providence, Rhode Island

Ronald S. Duman, Ph.D.
Professor, Departments of Psychiatry and Pharmacology, Yale University School of Medicine; and Laboratory of Molecular Psychiatry, Connecticut Mental Health Center, New Haven, Connecticut

Ronald P. Hammer Jr., Ph.D.
Professor, Departments of Psychiatry, Anatomy, Pharmacology and Neuroscience, Tufts University School of Medicine and Laboratory of Research in Psychiatry, New England Medical Center, Boston, Massachusetts

Stephan Heckers, M.D.
Assistant Professor, Department of Psychiatry, Harvard Medical School and Massachusetts General Hospital, Boston, Massachusetts

Donald C. Goff, M.D.
Associate Professor, Department of Psychiatry, Harvard Medical School and Massachusetts General Hospital, Boston, Massachusetts

Gary B. Kaplan, M.D.
Associate Professor, Departments of Psychiatry and Human Behavior and Molecular Pharmacology, Physiology and Biotechnology, Brown Medical School and Veterans Affairs Medical Center, Providence, Rhode Island

Justine M. Kent, M.D.
Assistant Professor, Department of Psychiatry, Columbia University College of Physicians and Surgeons and New York State Psychiatric Institute, New York, New York

Kimberly A. Leite-Morris, B.S.
Graduate Program, Department of Biochemistry, Microbiology, and Molecular Genetics, University of Rhode Island and Veterans Affairs Medical Center, Providence, Rhode Island

Gerard Marek, M.D., Ph.D.
Assistant Professor, Department of Psychiatry, Yale University School of Medicine; and Laboratory of Molecular Psychiatry, Connecticut Mental Health Center, New Haven, Connecticut

Ralph A. Nixon, M.D., Ph.D.
Professor, Departments of Psychiatry and Cell Biology, New York University School of Medicine; and Director, Center for Dementia Research, Nathan Kline Institute, Orangeburg, New York

Scott L. Rauch, M.D.
Associate Professor, Department of Psychiatry, Harvard Medical School, and Psychiatric Neuroimaging Research, Departments of Psychiatry and Radiology, Massachusetts General Hospital, Boston, Massachusetts

Stephen P. Salloway, M.D., M.S.
Associate Professor, Departments of Clinical Neurosciences and Psychiatry and Human Behavior, Brown Medical School; and Department of Neurology, Butler Hospital, Providence, Rhode Island

Roberto B. Sassi, M.D.
Postdoctoral Research Fellow, Western Psychiatric Institute and Clinic, University of Pittsburgh School of Medicine, Pittsburgh, Pennsylvania; and Department of Psychiatry, University of Sao Paulo School of Medicine, Sao Paulo, Brazil

Jair C. Soares, M.D.
Assistant Professor of Psychiatry, Western Psychiatric Institute and Clinic, University of Pittsburgh School of Medicine, Pittsburgh, Pennsylvania

Gregory M. Sullivan, M.D.
Assistant Professor, Department of Psychiatry, Columbia University College of Physicians and Surgeons and New York State Psychiatric Institute, New York, New York

Introduction to the Progress in Psychiatry Series

The Progress in Psychiatry Series is designed to capture in print the excitement that comes from assembling a diverse group of experts from various locations to examine in detail the newest information about a developing aspect of psychiatry. This series emerged as a collaboration between the American Psychiatric Association's (APA's) Scientific Program Committee and American Psychiatric Publishing, Inc. Great interest is generated by a number of the symposia presented each year at the APA annual meeting, and we realized that much of the information presented there, carefully assembled by people who are deeply immersed in a given area, would unfortunately not appear together in print. The symposia sessions at the annual meetings provide an unusual opportunity for experts who otherwise might not meet on the same platform to share their diverse viewpoints for a period of 3 hours. Some new themes are repeatedly reinforced and gain credence, whereas in other instances disagreements emerge, enabling the audience and now the reader to reach informed decisions about new directions in the field. The Progress in Psychiatry Series allows us to publish and capture some of the best of the symposia and thus provide an in-depth treatment of specific areas that might not otherwise be presented in broader review formats.

Psychiatry is, by nature, an interface discipline, combining the study of mind and brain, of individual and social environments, of the humane and the scientific. Therefore, progress in the field is rarely linear—it often comes from unexpected sources. Furthermore, new developments emerge from an array of viewpoints that do not necessarily provide immediate agreement but rather expert examination of the issues. We intend to present innovative ideas and data that will enable the reader to participate in this process.

We believe the Progress in Psychiatry Series will provide you with an opportunity to review timely, new information in specific fields of interest as they are developing. We hope you find that the excitement of the presentations is captured in the written word and that this book proves to be informative and enjoyable reading.

David Spiegel, M.D.
Series Editor
Progress in Psychiatry Series

Preface

Psychiatric disorders represent a complex interaction between psychological, developmental, neurobiological, and genetic factors. This book focuses on the neurobiological elements of psychiatric conditions. In the last 30 years, much has been learned about the neuroanatomic, neurophysiological, neurochemical, and molecular elements that contribute to major psychiatric illnesses such as schizophrenia, drug dependence, anxiety disorders, major depression, bipolar disorder, and dementias. In this book, we strive to integrate recent research findings about the neural circuitry and signaling pathways that influence the development and expression of psychiatric disorders. We attempt to present psychiatric neuroscience in a relatively brief and readable format. Our aim is to inform psychiatric clinicians as well as students of psychiatry, neuroscience, and psychopharmacology.

For clarity and consistency, each clinical chapter is organized into the following headings: Clinical Presentation, Neural Circuitry, Signaling Pathways, and Psychopharmacology. Emphasis is placed on the sections covering neuroanatomic (Neural Circuitry) and neurochemical and molecular (Signaling Pathways) mechanisms relating to each psychiatric disorder. To establish the framework for the material covered in these sections, we begin with two introductory chapters on signaling pathways and functional neural circuitry. Chapters on psychiatric disorders follow. We would like to express our appreciation to the chapter authors for their state-of-the-art presentations on the neurobiology of psychiatric disorders and also to Robert Emma for his expert graphical assistance provided for our cover design.

Our knowledge of psychiatric neuroscience has grown exponentially during the 1990s, appropriately termed "the decade of the brain." We believe that this book provides a bridge toward a better understanding of psychiatric illness, albeit just the start of a much longer quest. Nevertheless, this represents an important step in the right direction.

Gary B. Kaplan, M.D.
Ronald P. Hammer Jr., Ph.D.

CHAPTER 1

[handwritten margin note: middle tier, Thalamus, Basal ganglia, limbic]

Introduction to Functional Neural Circuitry

Stephen P. Salloway, M.D., M.S.
Ari Blitz, M.D.

In this chapter we introduce functional brain systems to provide a foundation for understanding the psychiatric disorders described in this book. Our modern concept of brain-behavior relationships began in the nineteenth century with Paul Broca's reports of nonfluent aphasia following infarction to the left lateral frontal lobe. These case reports and subsequent lesion studies gave rise to the view that specific brain structures carried out defined actions (e.g., Broca's area and motor speech). This view was followed by the evolution of the concept of the *limbic system,* an interconnected group of structures mediating emotion and complex behaviors. In 1985, Garrett Alexander, Mahlon DeLong, and Peter Strick described five distinct frontal-subcortical circuits contributing to the regulation of mood, personality, and cognition (Alexander et al. 1986). Marsel Mesulam and many cognitive neuroscientists have expanded on the concept of brain circuits by proposing the term *neural networks* to describe the pattern of activation in distributed brain regions involved in cognition and behavior (Mesulam 1990).

The brain is organized into three tiers: a lower tier, composed of the brain stem and cerebellum; a middle tier, containing the thalamus, basal ganglia, and many components of the limbic system; and an upper tier, consisting of the cortex (McLean 1970) (Figure 1–1). The brain stem regulates arousal, autonomic function, and internal states. The cell bodies for the key neurotransmitters that regulate behavior are found in the

---

This work was supported in part by the Howard Hughes Medical Institute–Medical Research Training Fellowships Program and by National Institute of Mental Health (NIMH) Grant K08MH01487.

1

upper brain stem. The middle tier modulates emotion and memory and helps control speed of movement and rate of thinking. The upper tier carries out higher-level sensory processing and is responsible for motor control, complex thought, and memory storage. In this chapter our focus is on the brain's middle tier, with special emphasis on the limbic system and the prefrontal-subcortical circuits that regulate behavior (Figure 1–2).

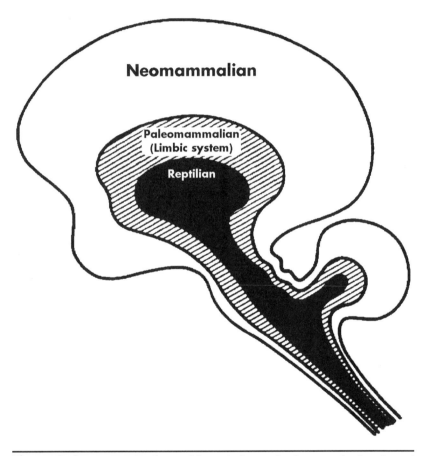

Figure 1–1. *McLean's schema of the evolutionary development of a three-layered triune brain. Note the location of the limbic system in the middle tier.*

Source. Reprinted from Mega MS, Cummings JL, Salloway S, et al.: "The Limbic System: An Anatomic, Phylogenetic, and Clinical Perspective." *Journal of Neuropsychiatry and Clinical Neurosciences* 9:315–330, 1997. Copyright 1997, American Psychiatric Press, Inc. Used with permission.

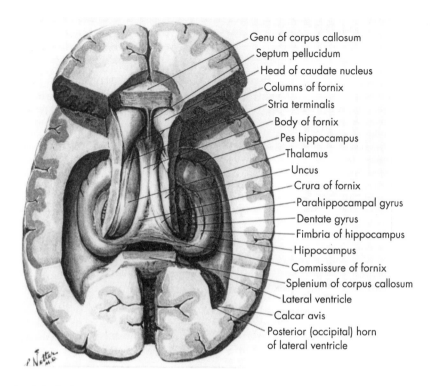

Genu of corpus callosum
Septum pellucidum
Head of caudate nucleus
Columns of fornix
Stria terminalis
Body of fornix
Pes hippocampus
Thalamus
Uncus
Crura of fornix
Parahippocampal gyrus
Dentate gyrus
Fimbria of hippocampus
Hippocampus
Commissure of fornix
Splenium of corpus callosum
Lateral ventricle
Calcar avis
Posterior (occipital) horn
of lateral ventricle

Figure 1–2. *Upper cortex and white matter tracts of the brain removed, revealing the close relationship of the limbic system (hippocampus and fornix) and striatum in the center of the brain.*

Source. Copyright 1983, Novartis. Reprinted with permission from *The Netter Collection of Medical Illustrations,* Vol. 1, Part I, illustrated by Frank H. Netter, M.D. All rights reserved.

We begin this chapter with an overview of how information about brain-behavior relationships is obtained. Cortical function is then illustrated, using visual processing as an example of specialized processing of sensory stimuli in different cortical regions. The remainder of the chapter highlights the functional organization of the limbic system, the prefrontal cortex, the frontal-subcortical-thalamic circuits, and the brain-stem systems that regulate behavior. Each section contains information on the location of the structures; their connections, neurochemistry, and primary functions; and the clinical syndromes associated with disease or injury to the system.

Approaches to Understanding Brain-Behavior Relationships

How do we obtain knowledge about functional brain circuits and systems? The roots of neuropsychiatry are strongly grounded in careful clinical observation and neuropathological correlation. The elegant histological sections of the nervous system produced by Ramón y Cajal and the new histological staining techniques introduced by Franz Nissl were instrumental in the development of Korbinian Brodmann's cytoarchitectonic map during the first decade of the twentieth century. These developments provided the foundation for clinical investigators such as Alois Alzheimer and Karl Wernicke to make important discoveries about the neuropathology of dementia and the brain regions responsible for different types of aphasia.

In animal models, advances in electrophysiology, such as single-unit recording, make it possible to study the electrical activity of individual neurons in real time in ambulatory subjects. Microdialysis devices can be placed in the limbic system in animals to monitor the chemical milieu at rest, during behavioral activation, or in disease states. Well-circumscribed lesions in specific structures can be made experimentally in laboratory animals, allowing for more tightly controlled study of the behavioral sequelae of lesions. Because anatomic relationships are highly conserved across species, these animal models have proved to be very useful in investigating neuroanatomic connections.

Standardized neuropsychological and behavioral techniques have been developed for assessing specific aspects of behavior and cognition. Normative data now exist, corrected for age and education level, for tests of memory, attention, visuospatial function, language, and executive function. Our understanding of functional relationships has also relied heavily on using these paradigms to study the behavioral effects of naturally occurring traumatic or ischemic lesions in individual patients. Unfortunately, naturally occurring lesions are often large and may incompletely involve several structures, which may make interpretation difficult.

Many advances in the understanding of brain-behavior relationships have come from the field of epilepsy surgery. Differential emotional and behavioral responses from each hemisphere are often observed during Amytal sodium infusion performed to test for language and memory in patients being screened for organic conditions such as epilepsy. Recordings from stereotactically placed intracranial microelectrodes taken to identify a seizure focus often provide valuable insights into behavioral and cognitive responses in specific brain regions.

In the early era of neuropsychiatry, clinicians and clinical researchers had to wait until autopsy to visualize the location and extent of brain pathology and to make a final diagnosis. Today, structural neuroimaging techniques such as computed tomography (CT) and magnetic resonance imaging (MRI) provide detailed views of neuroanatomy and neuropathology in the living patient with a high level of resolution. Volumetric structural imaging techniques can be used to monitor the natural evolution of brain changes in degenerative disorders such as Alzheimer's disease. These quantitative techniques can also be used to study aspects of brain development (e.g., the pattern and timing of neuronal migration and myelination).

Functional brain imaging has provided exciting new methods for studying brain-behavior relationships. The relationships between cerebral blood flow, metabolism, and behavior can be studied with positron emission tomography (PET), single photon emission computed tomography (SPECT), and functional magnetic resonance imaging (fMRI). Cognitive paradigms have been developed to probe brain activity during a variety of cognitive tasks in both healthy subjects and patients with specific brain disorders. For example, the brain areas activated when a subject generates a list of words or responds to fearful stimuli can be mapped. These techniques identify patterns of activation in the functional brain systems involved in completing a cognitive or behavioral task. Provocative stimuli can be used to study patterns of abnormal neuronal activity in psychiatric disorders—for example, measurement of blood flow and metabolism in patients with obsessive-compulsive disorder exposed to an object that elicits extreme anxiety. Magnetic resonance spectroscopy (MRS) can measure chemical constituents in specific brain regions to study the pathogenesis and progression of neuropsychiatric conditions.

Receptor ligand imaging can also be employed with PET and SPECT studies to study neurotransmitter systems in healthy and psychiatrically ill subjects. For example, ligands tagged with radioactive tracers can be used to examine dopaminergic activity in different stages of Parkinson's disease and cholinergic activity in Alzheimer's disease. Metabolic and ligand studies can be used to study pre- and postmedication neurochemical status in patients with psychiatric disorders, and findings may help identify patterns that predict treatment response.

Advances in neuropharmacology and molecular biology form much of the substance of the chapters that follow. These techniques allow us to dissect the neurochemical innervation of neuronal systems involved in regulating complex behaviors. Horseradish peroxidase and other staining techniques can detect retrograde and anterograde transport of specific neurotransmitters. Advances in receptor pharmacology provide essential information for refining our understanding of the neurochemistry of normal and disturbed behavior. For instance, we can study the integrity of receptor and postreceptor signaling systems in specific brain regions in postmortem tissue. One such example would be to compare the serotonergic system (including serotonin transporters, serotonin receptors, and serotonin-mediated second messengers) in prefrontal cortex tissue from patients with completed suicide and from control subjects.

The Cerebral Cortex

Functional Organization

The surface of the brain comprises the cerebral cortex, a thin layer of neurons that control movement, conscious experience, and higher-order cognitive function. Traditionally, the cortex is divided—somewhat arbitrarily—into four lobes: frontal, parietal, occipital, and temporal.

In most brain regions, the cortex encompasses six well-defined layers. The cortex consists of primary, secondary, and heteromodal functional areas. Primary cortical areas receive and perform initial processing of sensory or motor information (e.g., Brodmann area 17 in the occipital lobe for vision, Heschel's area in the superior temporal gyrus for hearing, the precentral gyrus for movement). Secondary association areas perform further processing of sensorimotor information within a specific modality (e.g., the visual association area in areas 18 and 19 in the parieto-occipital cortex and area 6 of the frontal cortex for supplementary motor function). Heteromodal association areas such as the prefrontal cortex integrate complex sensorimotor information from multiple modalities with motivational and affective states.

Neurons maintain corticocortical connections with neighboring neurons via small white matter bundles called U fibers. Longer, thicker fiber bundles connect lobes or hemispheres together (e.g., corpus callosum, uncinate fasciculus) or connect components of functional networks (e.g., cingulum bundle, fornix).

Cortical Processing of Visual Information

We begin our discussion of cortical function by reviewing how visual information is processed in different regions of the brain. Considerable progress has been made in understanding the cortical components of vision, which can serve as a model to apply to other complex sensory or motor modalities.

Visual information is transmitted by the optic nerve and optic tract from specific layers of the retina, the sensory organ, to the lateral geniculate nucleus of the thalamus, an important relay region in the brain. The lateral geniculate sends the information, via the optic radiations in the temporal and parietal cortex, to area 17 of the occipital lobe. Area 17 is located at the posteriormost portion of the occipital lobe and contains the cells that form the primary visual cortex, that region of the visual cortex with the most direct visual input and the simplest response properties. These cells also receive projections from corticocortical projections from neighboring higher-order visual areas. Cells in the primary visual cortex respond to a very small portion of the retina. The frequency with which they discharge action potentials increases or decreases in response to contrasts in light falling on the area of the retina for which they are responsible. That portion of the retina receives light from a single angle with respect to the pupil, which corresponds to a single location in visual space, known as the *receptive field* of the primary visual cortical neuron.

The primary visual cortex sends projections to, and receives projections from, numerous visual association areas. In these areas, cells respond to the presence of a line or movement in the receptive field of another area. As we examine visual areas farther away from the primary visual cortex, or indeed from other primary sensory areas, the response properties of the cells become more complex. Generally, the parietal association areas are spoken of as a location-related "where stream" of information, also referred to as the "dorsal stream" because projections extend from the primary visual cortex of the occipital lobe to the parietal lobe (Figure 1–3). In the dorsal stream, neurons are found to respond to the location of stimuli. In contrast, the association cortex of the temporal lobe is spoken of as a "what stream" or "ventral stream," its activity relating to the identity of an object apart from the object's location in space. Electrophysiological studies performed in ventral stream areas demonstrate a response to an object's identity (e.g., its color or shape) without regard to spatial information.

Visual information is further fed into the medial temporal lobe, amygdala, and hippocampus, where the emotional valence of objects is evaluated and where short-term memories of the visual experience are encoded (see "Limbic System" subsection, below). Additional processing of visual information takes place in the prefrontal cortex, where working memories for the appearance and location of the stimulus are encoded (see "Prefrontal Cortex" section, below).

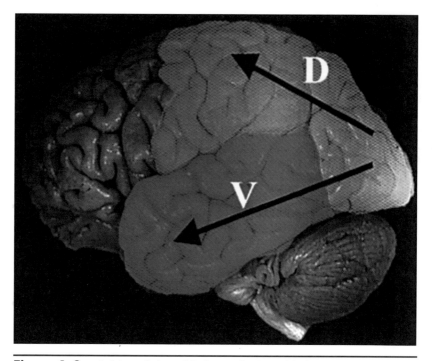

Figure 1–3. *Left lateral view of the human brain modified to show visual process-ing. Sensory information from the retina enters the primary visual sensory area in the occipital lobe (yellow) by way of a thalamic relay nucleus (not shown). Visual sensory information passes through a dorsal processing stream (D) involving association areas in the parietal lobe (red), which respond preferentially to an object's location. Sensory information also passes through a ventral processing stream (V) projecting to the tem-poral lobe (blue), which responds preferentially to an object's identity (color, shape, tex-ture) without regard to spatial information.*

Brain Systems Regulating Emotion and Behavior

Limbic System

A *limbus* is a margin or border, and the limbic system has come to en-compass a border between neurology and psychiatry. The term *limbic system* has become synonymous with the part of the brain that mediates emotional aspects of experience. Paul Broca first referred to the cingu-late gyrus, olfactory region, and hippocampus as the *grand lobe limbique* in 1878 (Figure 1–4A). Sanford Brown and Albert Schäfer reported in

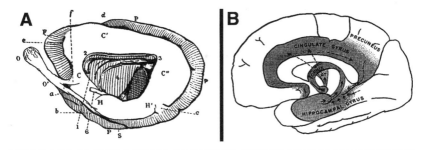

Figure 1–4. *A: "Le grand lobe limbique," common to all mammals, identified by Broca in 1878. B: The medial circuit of Papez, as depicted by McLean, was proposed in 1937 to support emotional processing.*

Source.   Reprinted from Mega MS, Cummings JL, Salloway S, et al.: "The Limbic System: An Anatomic, Phylogenetic, and Clinical Perspective." *Journal of Neuropsychiatry and Clinical Neurosciences* 9:315–330, 1997. Copyright 1997, American Psychiatric Press, Inc. Used with permission.

1888 that temporal lobectomy caused wild monkeys to be tame (Brown and Schäfer 1888). Heinrich Klüver and Paul Bucy later delineated the specific structures involved in producing this dramatic change in behavior (Klüver and Bucy 1939). In 1900, Wilhelm Bechterew found that lesions of the hippocampus, mammillary bodies, and anterior thalamus produced impairment in learning and memory. The histologist Ramón y Cajal described connections between the limbic lobe and the septal nuclei of the basal forebrain and between the hypothalamus and thalamus in the diencephalon.

In 1937, James Papez combined the results of anatomic studies with clinical reports of emotional disturbance following brain lesions to propose a circuit involved in the regulation of emotion. The Papez circuit includes the hippocampus, mammillary bodies, anterior nucleus of the thalamus, anterior cingulate gyrus, and cingulum bundle and their connections (Figure 1–4B). Paul Yakovlev stressed the importance of the orbitofrontal cortex, anterior temporal lobe, insula, amygdala, and dorsomedial thalamus in motivation and emotional expression (Yakovlev 1948). In 1949, Paul McLean linked the medial circuit of Papez with the basolateral structures of Yakovlev, referring to them for the first time as the *limbic system* (McLean 1949, 1970). Today, the definition of the limbic system has expanded to include the amygdala and entorhinal cortex in the medial temporal lobe, the septal nucleus at the base of the frontal lobe, the anterior cingulate gyrus, and the orbitofrontal cortex. The limbic system plays a key role in memory, cognition, mood and anxiety, social behavior, and regulation of drives and impulses.

Marsel Mesulam described two paralimbic belts, an archicortical belt with the hippocampus as its center and a paleocortical olfactory orbitofrontal belt closely associated with the amygdala (Mesulam 1985). The hippocampal-cingulate division conducts explicit sensory processing, enabling the conscious encoding of experience. The amygdalarorbitofrontal division examines the internal relevance of sensory stimuli and integrates affects, drives, and object associations. The two paralimbic divisions work in concert to integrate thought, feeling, and action (Figure 1–5).

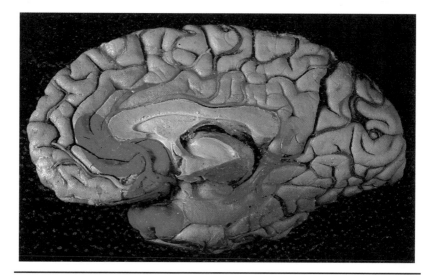

Figure 1–5. *Sagittal view of the brain, demonstrating the paralimbic trends of evolutionary cortical development. The phylogenetically older paralimbic amygdalarorbitofrontal belt* **(red)**, *involved in emotional processing, extends into the subcallosal cingulate, temporal polar region, and the anterior insula (not shown). The more recent hippocampal-centered belt* **(blue)**, *involved in learning and memory processing, extends its wave of cortical development dorsally through the posterior and anterior cingulate.*

Source. Adapted from Mega and Cummings 1997 and reprinted from Mega MS, Cummings JL, Salloway S, et al.: "The Limbic System: An Anatomic, Phylogenetic, and Clinical Perspective." *Journal of Neuropsychiatry and Clinical Neurosciences* 9:315–330, 1997. Copyright 1997, American Psychiatric Press, Inc. Used with permission.

Hippocampal-Cingulate Division and Cognitive Processing

The hippocampus, meaning "sea horse" (so named because of its shape), is composed of a three-layer archicortex and is located beneath the parahippocampal gyrus. The entorhinal cortex, surrounding the hippocampus on its inferomedial surface, contains a perforant pathway that serves as a gateway bringing information into the hippocampus. The hippocampus is divided into four regions, CA1–CA4, that surround the dentate gyrus (Figure 1–6). The main outflow tract for the hippocampus is a thick white matter bundle called the *fornix* (see Figure 1–2). The fornix connects the hippocampus to the septal nuclei in the base of the frontal lobe and to the mammillary bodies in the posterior hypothalamus.

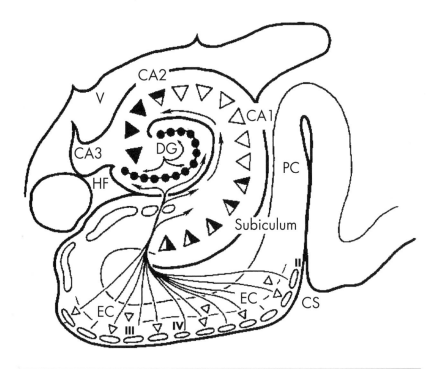

Figure 1–6. *Schematic coronal view showing cortical input to the hippocampus and entorhinal cortex. Direct cortical input to the hippocampal pyramidal neurons (CA1–CA3) and dentate gyrus granule cells (DG) is received via the perforant pathway that arises from the entorhinal cortex (EC). HF = hippocampal fissure; V = ventricle; PC = perirhinal cortex; CS = collateral sulcus.*

Source. Reprinted from Van Hoesen GW: "Ventromedial Temporal Lobe Anatomy, With Comments on Alzheimer's Disease and Temporal Injury." *Journal of Neuropsychiatry and Clinical Neurosciences* 9:331–341, 1997. Copyright 1997, American Psychiatric Press, Inc. Used with permission.

The hippocampus is involved in new learning, formation of episodic memories, spatial memory, orientation, and regulation of mood. The right hippocampus is specialized for spatial memory and the left hippocampus is dominant for verbal memory. The hippocampus contains local glutamatergic and GABAergic (i.e., activated by or secreting γ-aminobutyric acid [GABA]) circuits and is richly innervated by neurons from cholinergic, dopaminergic, noradrenergic, and serotonergic tracts.

The hippocampus is frequently involved in partial complex seizures and is often the site of the seizure focus in patients with behavioral disturbance due to temporal lobe epilepsy. In herpes varicella encephalitis, the hippocampus is often affected. The hippocampus is sensitive to anoxic injury, which produces confusion and amnesia.

The role of the hippocampus in the formation of episodic memories was highlighted by the famous case of H.M., who lost his ability to form new memories following bilateral hippocampectomy for refractory epilepsy (Milner 1972). The entorhinal cortex degenerates early in Alzheimer's disease, and the hippocampus is a site of heavy plaque and tangle formation (Killiany et al. 2000). Histological abnormalities have also been reported in the hippocampus and entorhinal cortex in schizophrenia and autism.

Amygdala and Emotional Processing

The amygdala ("almond") lies anterior and medial to the hippocampus. It consists of a cluster of nuclei divided into basolateral and corticomedial divisions. The basolateral region of the amygdala receives major input from the visual system and other sensory modalities. The amygdala has been referred to as the *valence center* because it attaches affective color and social meaning to sensory information. It also receives primary olfactory afferents from the lateral olfactory stria, which accounts for the major role that olfaction plays in emotion and behavior, especially in lower animals.

The amygdala has rich reciprocal connections with the orbitofrontal cortex. The amygdala connects to the basal forebrain cholinergic neurons in the septal nucleus via the stria terminalis and to hypothalamic and brain-stem autonomic areas via the ventral amygdalofugal pathway (Figure 1–7). It also connects to the nucleus accumbens in the ventral striatum via the extended amygdala. The extended amygdala plays a role in attaching emotional content to stimuli associated with drugs of abuse.

The amygdala plays a key role in the startle reflex and can generate fight-or-flight responses. The amygdala also helps regulate appetite, mood, aggression, sexual and social behavior, and comprehension of social cues. Rare cases of bilateral amygdala degeneration have been reported in which individuals cannot recognize fear in others, although

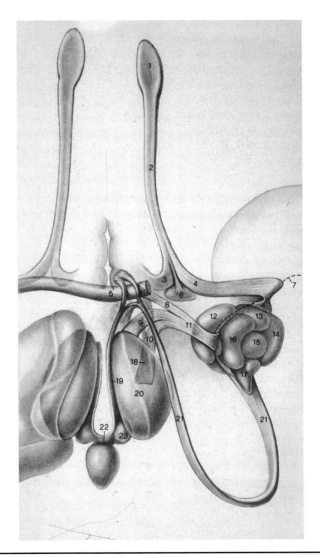

Figure 1–7. *Schema depicting dorsal view of connections of the amygdala: 1–4 = olfactory structures, 5 = anterior commissure, 6 = olfactory tubercle, 7 = limen insulae, 8 = diagonal band of Broca, 9 = inferior thalamic peduncle, 10 = medial telencephalic fasciculus, 11 = ventral amygdalofugal pathway, 12–17 = amygdaloid nuclei, 18 = lateral hypothalamic area, 19–20 = nucleus and stria medullaris, 21 = stria terminalis, 22 = habenular commissure, and 23 = septal nuclei.*

they are capable of feeling fear themselves (Tranel and Hyman 1990). Auras from partial seizures arising in the amygdala can cause olfactory sensations (e.g., odd smells like burning rubber), autonomic sensations (e.g., gnawing in the stomach; racing heart), automatic behaviors (e.g., picking at clothing), or psychic experiences (e.g., déjà vu, dreamy states, depersonalization, hallucinations, waves of fear). Many of these symptoms may be present during panic attacks.

The amygdala and overlying parahippocampal gyrus receive rich noradrenergic innervation from the locus coeruleus in the pons. These structures have been implicated in panic disorder. Surgical bilateral amygdalectomies for refractory epilepsy or aggression have produced the Klüver-Bucy syndrome. This syndrome causes individuals to be placid. Hyperorality is prominent; patients with this syndrome may attempt to eat nonfood items. Animals with the syndrome may fail to recognize dominant animals and may even initiate sex with animals from other species.

The amygdala also plays an important role in forming emotional memories. Emotionally arousing experiences tend to be well remembered. Extensive evidence indicates that stress-released adrenal hormones—epinephrine and cortisol—regulate the strength of emotional memory. These hormones act on the amygdala to enhance the storage of recent experiences. Lesions of the amygdala and β-blocking drugs block the memory-enhancing effects of emotional arousal, whereas infusion of norepinephrine in the amygdala enhances emotional memory (McGaugh et al. 1996). Posttraumatic stress disorder may represent a hyperactivation of this system.

Prefrontal Cortex

The frontal lobe, the largest lobe in the brain, takes up approximately one-third of the total cortical area. The frontal lobe can be divided into three sections. The first, occupying the precentral gyrus, is the primary motor cortex, and the second, lying just anterior to it, is the premotor cortex. Conscious movements are mediated in the primary motor cortex; the planning of complex actions occurs in the premotor cortex. The third area, and the one of greatest interest for psychiatry, is the prefrontal cortex. The prefrontal cortex is the portion of the frontal cortex lying anterior to the premotor and primary motor cortices (Figure 1–8). The prefrontal cortex can be been divided into three regions: 1) the executive prefrontal cortex, occupying the dorsal and lateral aspects of the prefrontal cortex; 2) the paralimbic prefrontal cortex, occupying the orbital and medial aspects of the prefrontal cortex; and 3) the anterior cingulate area.

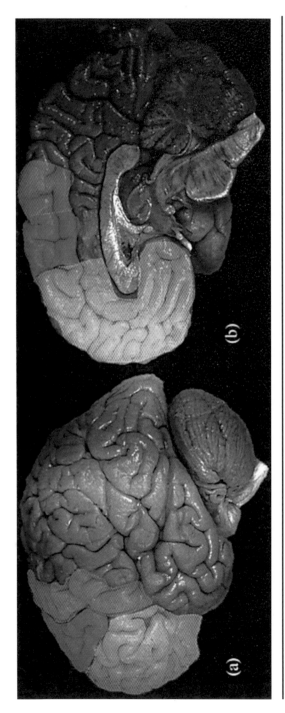

Figure 1–8. *Functional divisions of the frontal lobe of the human brain: A: Lateral view. B: Sagittal view. Primary motor cortex (red), premotor cortex (blue), and prefrontal cortex (yellow) are highlighted.*

Executive/Dorsolateral Prefrontal Cortex

The dorsolateral prefrontal cortex is responsible for executive aspects of cognition. It is here that the dorsal and ventral streams of information previously mentioned rejoin. The dorsolateral prefrontal cortex receives innervation from both the parietal and the temporal association cortices. The dorsolateral prefrontal cortex projects to the premotor cortex lying just posterior to it, suggesting its role in the transformation of sensory information into preparation for movement.

Executive functions involve integration of sensorimotor information from multiple modalities and formulation of behavioral responses. The dorsolateral prefrontal cortex has been implicated in executive functions such as cognitive speed and flexibility, task sequencing, higher-order attention, and working memory. These cognitive abilities allow us to complete the many complex daily tasks that are required to maintain an independent lifestyle. Barry Fogel and Paul Malloy have suggested that executive dysfunction may be a major cause of disability both in normal aging and in degenerative disorders such as Alzheimer's disease (Cahn-Weiner et al. 2000; Fogel 1994).

Lesions of sections of the dorsolateral prefrontal cortex in lower primates produce impairment in spatial working memory (Funahashi et al. 1989). In the spatial delayed matching–to–sample task, the subject is shown an object placed randomly in one of several positions in space. The object disappears, and after a delay, the subject must indicate the location at which the object previously appeared. Lesioned subjects are able to perform the task only when no delay is interposed or when only recognition of the object's identity is required. Using single-cell recording, Patricia Goldman-Rakic identified individual neurons in the dorsolateral prefrontal cortex that commence firing at the beginning of the delay period and maintain their activity until a response regarding location of the object is demanded. Structural or neurochemical interference with these specialized neurons produces impairment of spatial working memory (Goldman-Rakic 1994).

The ability to maintain information in working memory has important implications. It has been suggested that the primary defect in schizophrenia may lie in the dorsolateral prefrontal cortex, rendering patients unable to maintain information in working memory. Indeed, a version of the delayed matching–to–sample task in human subjects demonstrated a deficit for schizophrenic patients similar in kind to that observed in experimental animals with dorsolateral prefrontal lesions (Goldman-Rakic 1994). Impairments in dorsolateral prefrontal cortical activation during the Wisconsin Card Sorting Test (a measure of executive cognition requiring the shifting of set in response to environmental stimuli) are a consistent finding in schizophrenia. This deficit provides further evidence for functional impairment in the dorsolateral prefrontal cortex in the disorder (Weinberger et al. 1994).

Paralimbic/Orbitofrontal Cortex

The orbitofrontal cortex, that portion of the prefrontal cortex lying on the *medial* and *orbital* (literally, "above the orbit") surfaces of the hemisphere, has come to be regarded as an extension of the limbic system. It is involved in complex aspects of human behavior, such as regulation of impulses, mood, and personality. The orbitofrontal cortex receives innervation from the mediodorsal nucleus of the thalamus, which in turn receives input from almost all other cortical structures. The orbitofrontal cortex has reciprocal connections to the amygdala both through the ventral amygdalofugal tract and through the stria terminalis. These connections carry efferent signals to the mediodorsal nucleus and through the uncinate fasciculus, which travels directly from the temporal lobe to the frontal lobe. These pathways provide the orbitofrontal cortex with access to all information necessary to respond to the environment with respect to the motivational and cognitive state of the individual.

The orbitofrontal cortex is a common site for closed-head injury. Patients with damage confined to the ventromedial prefrontal cortex demonstrate mood lability, disinhibition, impulsivity, inappropriate behavior, disrupted social relationships, and impaired judgment (Damasio et al. 1990; Harrington et al. 1997; Tranel 1997).

Dysfunction in the orbitofrontal cortex has been implicated in a number of psychiatric disorders. Patients with obsessive-compulsive disorder have demonstrated hyperactivity in the orbitofrontal cortex in SPECT and PET studies using tracers to measure blood flow and metabolic activity. The hyperactivity in the orbitofrontal area normalizes following successful treatment (Baxter 1992). Helen Mayberg found hypoactivity in the orbitofrontal cortex of patients with secondary depression (Mayberg 1994).

Anterior Cingulate Gyrus

The cingulate gyrus spans the medial surface of the brain from the prefrontal cortex to the parieto-occipital junction, providing a bridge between the systems performing emotional, cognitive, motor, and sensory processing. The anterior cingulate gyrus contains segments in the subcallosal region anterior to the genu and above the corpus callosum (see Figure 1–5). The anterior cingulate is involved in attention, drive, motivation, memory, and initiation of speech.

The subcallosal segment is closely allied with the amygdalar-orbitofrontal portion of the limbic system involved in emotional processing. The anterior cingulate is closely connected to the nucleus accumbens and is an important component of reward systems in the brain. Area 24 in the anterior cingulate gyrus is a nexus in the distributed networks that regulate internal motivating states and externally directed attention. This segment anterior to the genu is a transition zone between emotional and cognitive limbic circuits. Robust connections with the sensory processing region of the posterior cingulate overlap with rich reciprocal amygdalar connections. Area 24 is also strongly connected to the dorsolateral prefrontal cortex, which modulates executive function. Mayberg has suggested that metabolic activity in area 24 might be used as a marker for treatment response in depression. Depressed subjects with high metabolic activity in this region were more likely than those without such activity to respond to antidepressant medication (Mayberg 1997). The supracallosal segment of the anterior cingulate is closely connected to the hippocampus via the cingulum bundle and the posterior cingulate gyrus and is involved in short-term memory and higher-order attention.

Lesions to the anterior cingulate most commonly cause apathy. Bilateral injury to the anterior cingulate can produce a condition of akinetic mutism in which the person is alert but has tremendous inertia, with little spontaneous movement or speech. The anterior cingulate has rich dopaminergic inputs, and patients with apathy and akinetic mutism sometimes improve with dopamine agonists and stimulants such as methylphenidate (Ross and Stewart 1981). Patients with obsessive-compulsive disorder may also demonstrate hyperactivity in the anterior cingulate gyrus on functional imaging studies. Cingulotomies (small cuts in the cingulum bundle) are still occasionally used for the treatment of refractory depression, pain, and obsessive-compulsive disorder.

Basal Ganglia and Ventral Striatum

The striatum consists of the caudate and the putamen. These structures are histologically similar and are separated by thick bands of fibers traveling in the internal capsule. When dissected, the overlapping areas of caudate, putamen, and internal capsule give the appearance of being striated, or striped. The more dorsal components of the striatum are associated with the extrapyramidal system and motor control. The more ventral areas are involved in motivation, cognition, and emotion. At their ventralmost extent, the caudate and putamen appear to merge into a single structure, called the *nucleus accumbens* (Figure 1–9A).

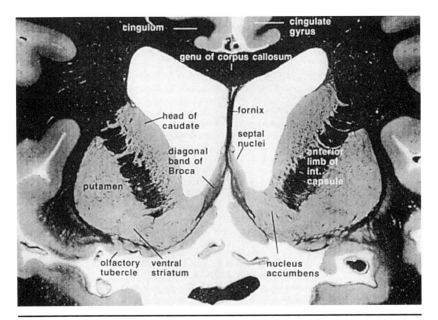

Figure 1–9A. *Weigert-stained coronal view of the ventral striatum and nucleus accumbens, shown at the level of the frontal horns of the lateral ventricle.*

Source. Adapted from DeArmond SJ, Fusco MM, Dewey MM: *Structure of the Human Brain: A Photographic Atlas,* 2nd Edition. New York, Oxford University Press, 1976; and reprinted from Salloway S, Cummings J: "Subcortical Disease and Neuropsychiatric Illness." *Journal of Neuropsychiatry and Clinical Neurosciences* 6:93–99, 1994. Copyright 1994, American Psychiatric Press, Inc. Used with permission from both publications.

The striatum is composed of acetylcholinesterase-poor patches (striosomes) rich in opiate receptors and surrounded by an acetylcholinesterase-rich matrix. Striosomes have high levels of D_1 receptors and prominent limbic input. The matrix is rich in D_2 receptors with close connections to the substantia nigra. The striosomes are thought to be mostly involved in cognitive and behavioral processing, whereas the matrix is a major component of the extrapyramidal motor system.

The ventral caudate, ventral putamen, ventral pallidum, nucleus accumbens, and olfactory tubercle form the ventral striatum. The ventral striatum receives inputs from the ventral tegmental area of the midbrain and projects to the dorsomedial nucleus of the thalamus and the prefrontal cortex to regulate cognition and motivated behaviors. Parallel circuits from the midbrain-striatum-pallidum-thalamus-frontal lobe that use similar neurotransmitters exist for extrapyramidal and cognitive behavior (Graybiel 1990; Nauta 1986) (Figure 1–9B).

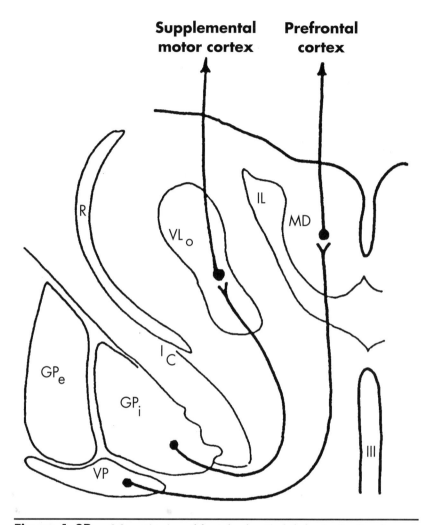

Figure 1–9B. *Schematic view of frontal-subcortical-thalamic circuits, shown at the level of the pallidum and thalamus. The extrapyramidal motor circuit involves the globus pallidus interna (GP$_i$) and ventral lateral nucleus of the thalamus (VL$_o$) and connects to the supplementary motor cortex. The related circuit of the ventral striatum involves the ventral pallidum (VP) and mediodorsal nucleus of the thalamus (MD) and connects to the prefrontal cortex. I$_C$ = internal capsule; III = third ventricle; R = reticular nucleus of the thalamus; GP$_e$ = globus pallidus externa.*

Source.   Reprinted from Nauta HJ: "The Relationship of the Basal Ganglia to the Limbic System," in *Handbook of Clinical Neurology,* Vol. 5: Extrapyramidal Disorders. Edited by Vinken PJ, Bruyn GW, Klawans HL. New York, Elsevier Science, 1986, pp. 19–29. Copyright 1986, Elsevier Science. Used with permission.

The nucleus accumbens sits at the crossroads of the limbic system, extrapyramidal motor system, and basal forebrain. The accumbens is divided into a core and a shell (Figure 1–10). The core contains striosomes and a matrix resembling the striatum and is embryologically and functionally connected to the striatum. The shell's margins blur into the olfactory tubercle and extended amygdala. The shell receives limbic inputs and has rich dopaminergic inputs from the ventral tegmental area (Heimer et al. 1997). The nucleus accumbens shell, a major node for reward systems in the brain, is a primary site for the action of cocaine and other drugs of abuse.

Frontal-Subcortical Circuits

The prefrontal cortex is connected to the striatum and thalamus by distinct circuits that help regulate behavior. The circuits consist of projections extending from a specific region of the prefrontal cortex to the head of the caudate, the globus pallidus, and the medial thalamus and back to the prefrontal cortex (Figure 1–11). Three distinct prefrontal-subcortical-thalamic behavioral circuits have been identified: 1) the dorsolateral prefrontal circuit, which mediates executive cognition; 2) the orbital-prefrontal circuit, which regulates impulses and mood; and 3) the anterior cingulate circuit, which modulates drive and motivation. Figure 1–12 shows the subcortical connections of these three circuits.

The frontal lobe sends excitatory glutamatergic fibers to the striatum. The striatal projections to the globus pallidus and the pallidal connections to the thalamus are GABAergic. The thalamic inputs back to the frontal lobe are glutamatergic. Another important indirect pathway extends between the globus pallidus (GABAergic) and the subthalamic nucleus and back to the globus pallidus (glutamatergic). The motor striatum also receives dopaminergic inputs from the substantia nigra pars compacta, and the ventral striatum receives strong dopaminergic inputs from the ventral tegmental area. These additional inputs, together with limbic connections to the basal ganglia, constitute the distributed networks that regulate many behaviors. Moreover, the interaction between neurotransmitters in these intersecting circuits is quite complex: each neuron contains receptors for multiple neurotransmitters, and cells express important neuromodulators such as substance P and neurotensin.

Diencephalon and Brain Stem

The hypothalamus is composed of many nuclei that regulate mood, complex behaviors, and cognition. The mammillary bodies are the most

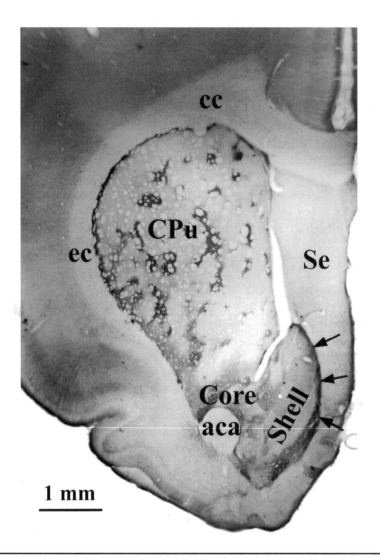

Figure 1–10. *Photomicrograph of a section through the rat striatum showing the shell and core of the nucleus accumbens inferomedial to the caudate/putamen (CPu). The shell contains a high density of opiate receptors. Note the intense μ opiate receptor antibody staining (**dark band**) along the medial edge of the shell of the accumbens (**arrows**) and the dark-stained patches and subcallosal streak in the striatum. aca = anterior limb of the internal capsule; cc = corpus callosum; ec = external capsule; Se = septum.*

Source.   Reprinted from Heimer L, Alheid GF, de Olmos JS, et al.: "The Accumbens: Beyond the Core-Shell Dichotomy." *Journal of Neuropsychiatry and Clinical Neurosciences* 9:354–381, 1997. Copyright 1997, American Psychiatric Press, Inc. Used with permission.

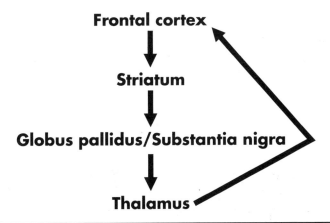

Figure 1–11. *Schematic outline of frontal-subcortical-thalamic circuits involved in regulating behavior.*

posterior nuclei of the hypothalamus. They receive input from the hippocampus-fornix and send output to the anterior nucleus of the thalamus via the mammillo-thalamic tract. As a result, they are a key component of the Papez limbic memory circuit. Injury to the mammillary bodies can cause anterograde memory impairment, such as that seen in the Wernicke-Korsakoff syndrome due to thiamine deficiency in alcoholism. Wernicke-Korsakoff syndrome is also associated with confabulation and psychosis.

Stimulation of the lateral nucleus of the hypothalamus induces aggressive behavior, increased sexual activity, and voracious eating. Infusion of acetylcholine in the lateral nucleus also elicits aggression and sham rage. In contrast, stimulation of the ventral posteromedial nucleus of the hypothalamus induces satiety and cessation of eating, with animals showing placid behavior. Individuals with lesions in this nucleus exhibit poor control of aggression.

The suprachiasmatic nucleus regulates circadian rhythm. Dysfunction in the suprachiasmatic nucleus, a common feature of Alzheimer's disease, causes dysregulation of the day-night sleep cycle. Sleep disturbance, agitation, disturbed appetite, and memory impairment are common symptoms associated with major depression, suggesting involvement of the hypothalamus in that disorder as well.

The primary cell bodies for the monoamine and cholinergic neurotransmitters that regulate behavior are located in the brain stem and the basal forebrain. The principal cell bodies for dopamine are found in the anterior portion of the midbrain in the substantia nigra and ventral tegmental area (Figure 1–13). Dopaminergic neurons in the substantia

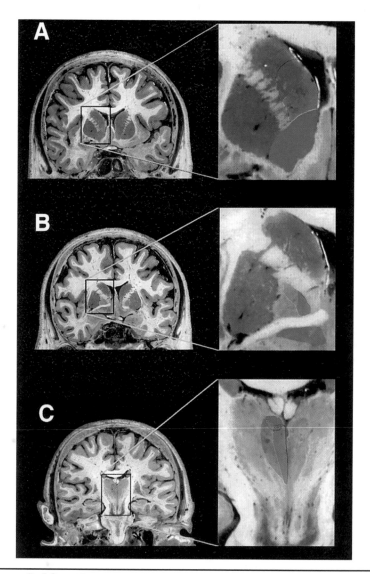

Figure 1–12. *The anatomy of the frontal subcortical circuits illustrates the general segregated anatomy of the following: dorsolateral (**blue**), orbitofrontal (**green**), and anterior cingulate (**red**) circuits in the striatum (**A**), pallidum (**B**), and mediodorsal thalamus (**C**).*

Source. Reprinted from Mega MS, Cummings JL, Salloway S, et al.: "The Limbic System: An Anatomic, Phylogenetic, and Clinical Perspective." *Journal of Neuropsychiatry and Clinical Neurosciences* 9:315–330, 1997. Copyright 1997, American Psychiatric Press, Inc. Used with permission.

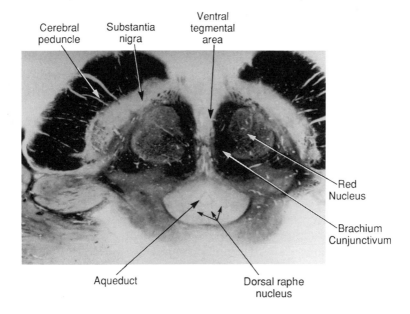

Cerebral peduncle

Substantia nigra

Ventral tegmental area

Red Nucleus

Brachium Cunjunctivum

Aqueduct

Dorsal raphe nucleus

Figure 1–13. *Section of the midbrain shown with Weigert stain for myelin (**black areas**). The principal dopaminergic cell bodies are located in the substantia nigra and ventral tegmental area in the anterior midbrain. The primary cell bodies for serotonin are located in the dorsal raphe surrounding the cerebral aqueduct.*

nigra innervate the striatum, primarily via D_2 dopamine receptors, and play a major role in modulating the extrapyramidal motor system. Dopaminergic neurons in the ventral tegmental area innervate the prefrontal cortex, ventral striatum, and medial temporal lobe. These neurons synapse on different dopamine receptor subtypes and mediate mood, drive, cognitive speed, and emotion. Prominent inputs from the ventral tegmental area into the nucleus accumbens play a central role in regulating the rewarding and motivational effects of drugs of abuse.

The primary cell bodies for serotonin are found in the dorsal raphe of the posterior midbrain just anterior to the cerebral aqueduct (see Figure 1–13). Serotonergic neurons innervate the striatum and cortex diffusely, with inputs to the frontal lobe, medial temporal lobe, basal ganglia, and ventral striatum as well as to other areas of the cortex, the brain stem, the cerebellum, and the spinal cord. Serotonin is involved in regulation of mood, sleep, pain, anxiety, motor tone, vasoconstriction, and pleasure.

The primary cell bodies for acetylcholine are found in the basal forebrain (see Figure 1–9A). Cholinergic neurons in the septal nucleus provide rich projections to the hippocampus and medial temporal lobe, and neurons from the nucleus basalis of Meynert and the diagonal band of Broca innervate the cerebral cortex. Loss of cholinergic neurons occurs early in Alzheimer's disease, causing short-term memory impairment. Forebrain cholinergic neurons also participate in attention, motivation, and emotional processing. Treatment with cholinesterase inhibitors can sometimes improve apathy, irritability, and attentional problems in Alzheimer's disease.

The primary cell bodies for norepinephrine are found in the locus coeruleus in the dorsal rostral pons. These neurons project to the striatum, the amygdala and limbic system, the prefrontal cortex, and other cortical areas. Noradrenergic neurons participate in arousal, sleep induction, anxiety, and autonomic activity. Dysfunction in the noradrenergic inputs to the limbic cortex is probably a major component underlying panic episodes. The noradrenergic system is also a target in treatment of attention-deficit/hyperactivity disorder and depression.

Conclusions

Caution is advised in applying too literally even such benign concepts as the neural circuit toward an understanding of brain function. It must be realized that the actual connections of the brain are too numerous and too varied to submit fully to such simplification. Our approach in this chapter has been to simplify somewhat the current state of knowledge in an attempt to create a framework that will hold the more detailed clinical information presented in later chapters.

The functional systems that regulate behavior are currently the focus of intense research activity, and the models presented here are continually evolving. Understanding the neurochemistry and functions of the different components within each system and the complex interactions between systems is the primary focus of modern neuroscience. The reader should use this information as a template that can be modified as new information becomes available.

References

Alexander GE, DeLong MR, Strick PL: Parallel organization of functionally segregated circuits linking basal ganglia and cortex. Ann Rev Neurosci 9:357–381, 1986

Baxter LR Jr: Neuroimaging studies of obsessive compulsive disorder. Psychiatr Clin North Am 15:871–884, 1992

Bechterew W: Demonstration eines gehirns mit Zestörung der vorderen und inneren Theile der Hirnrinde beider Schläfenlappen [Demonstration of a brain with the frontal portion of the skull damaged]. Neurologisches Centralblatt 20:990–991, 1900

Broca P: Anatomie comparée des circonvolutions cérébrales: le grand lobe limbique et la scissure limbique dans la série des mammifères [Anatomic comparison of cerebral convolutions: the great limbic lobe and limbic sulci in a series of mammals]. Revue d'Anthropologie 1:384–498, 1878

Brown S, Schäfer EA: An investigation into the functions of the occipital and temporal lobes of the monkey's brain. Philos Trans R Soc Lond 179:303–327, 1888

Cahn-Weiner DA, Malloy PF, Boyle PA, et al: Prediction of functional status from neuropsychological tests in community-dwelling elderly individuals. Clin Neuropsychol 14:187–195, 2000

Damasio AR, Tranel D, Damasio H: Individuals with sociopathic behavior caused by frontal damage fail to respond autonomically to social stimuli. Behav Brain Res 41:81–94, 1990

DeArmond SJ, Fusco MM, Dewey MM: Structure of the Human Brain: A Photographic Atlas, 2nd Edition. New York, Oxford University Press, 1976

Fogel BS: The significance of frontal system disorders for medical practice and health policy. J Neuropsychiatry Clin Neurosci 6:343–346, 1994

Funahashi S, Bruce CJ, Goldman-Rakic PS: Mnemonic coding of visual space in the monkey's dorsolateral prefrontal cortex. J Neurophysiol 61:331–349, 1989

Goldman-Rakic PS: Working memory dysfunction in schizophrenia. J Neuropsychiatry Clin Neurosci 6:348–357, 1994

Graybiel AM: Neurotransmitters and neuromodulators in the basal ganglia. Trends Neurosci 13:224–253, 1990

Harrington C, Salloway S, Malloy P: Dramatic neurobehavioral disorder in two cases following anteromedial frontal lobe injury, delay psychosis and marked change in personality. Neurocase 3:137–149, 1997

Heimer L, Alheid GF, de Olmos JS, et al: The accumbens: beyond the core-shell dichotomy. J Neuropsychiatry Clin Neurosci 9:354–381, 1997

Killiany RJ, Gomez-Isla T, Moss M, et al: Use of structural magnetic resonance imaging to predict who will get Alzheimer's disease. Ann Neurol 47:430–439, 2000

Klüver H, Bucy PC: Preliminary analysis of functions of the temporal lobes in monkeys. Archives of Neurology and Psychiatry 42:979–1000, 1939

Mayberg HS: Frontal lobe dysfunction in secondary depression. J Neuropsychiatry Clin Neurosci 6:428–442, 1994

Mayberg HS: Limbic-cortical dysregulation: a proposed model of depression. J Neuropsychiatry Clin Neurosci 9:471–481, 1997

McGaugh JL, Cahill L, Roozendaal B: Involvement of the amygdala in memory storage: interaction with other brain systems. Proc Natl Acad Sci U S A 93:13508–13514, 1996

McLean PD: Psychosomatic disease and the "visceral brain": recent developments bearing on the Papez theory of emotion. Psychosom Med 11:338–353, 1949

McLean PD: The triune brain, emotion and scientific bias, in The Neurosciences: Second Study Program. Edited by Schmitt FO. New York, Rockefeller University Press, 1970, pp 336–349

Mega MS, Cummings JL: The cingulate and cingulate syndromes, in Contemporary Behavioral Neurology. Edited by Trimble MR, Cummings JL. Boston, MA, Butterworth-Heinemann, 1997, pp 189–214

Mega MS, Cummings JL, Salloway S, et al: The limbic system: an anatomic, phylogenetic, and clinical perspective. J Neuropsychiatry Clin Neurosci 9:315–330, 1997

Mesulam M-M: Patterns in behavioral neuroanatomy: association areas, the limbic system, and hemispheric specialization, in Principles of Behavioral Neurology. Edited by Mesulam M-M. Philadelphia, PA, FA Davis, 1985, pp 1–70

Mesulam M-M: Large-scale neurocognitive networks and distributed processing for attention, language, and memory. Ann Neurol 28:597–613, 1990

Milner B: Disorders of learning and memory after temporal lobe lesions in man. Clin Neurosurg 19:421–446, 1972

Nauta HJ: The relationship of the basal ganglia to the limbic system, in Handbook of Clinical Neurology, Vol 5: Extrapyramidal Disorders. Edited by Vinken PJ, Bruyn GW, Klawans HL. New York, Elsevier, 1986, pp 19–29

Netter FH: The Netter Collection of Medical Illustrations. East Hanover, NJ, Novartis Pharmaceuticals Corp, 1997

Nieuwenhuys R, Voogd J, van Huijzen C: The Human Central Nervous System, 3rd Edition. New York, Springer-Verlag, 1988

Papez JW: A proposed mechanism of emotion. Archives of Neurology and Psychiatry 38:725–743, 1937

Ross ED, Stewart RM: Akinetic mutism from hypothalamic damage: successful treatment with dopamine agonists. Neurology 31:1435–1439, 1981

Salloway S, Cummings J: Subcortical disease and neuropsychiatric illness. J Neuropsychiatry Clin Neurosci 6:93–99, 1994

Tranel D: Functional neuroanatomy: neuropsychological correlates of cortical and subcortical damage, in The American Psychiatric Press Textbook of Neuropsychiatry, 3rd Edition. Edited by Yudofsky SC, Hales RE. Washington, DC, American Psychiatric Press, 1997, pp 77–120

Tranel D, Hyman BT: Neuropsychological correlates of bilateral amygdala damage. Arch Neurol 47:349–355, 1990

Van Hoesen GW: Ventromedial temporal lobe anatomy, with comments on Alzheimer's disease and temporal injury. J Neuropsychiatry Clin Neurosci 9:331–341, 1997

Weinberger DR, Aloia MS, Goldberg TE, et al: The frontal lobes and schizophrenia. J Neuropsychiatry Clin Neurosci 6:419–427, 1994

Yakovlev PI: Motility, behavior, and the brain. J Nerv Ment Dis 107:313–335, 1948

CHAPTER 2

Introduction to Neuronal Signaling Pathways

Gary B. Kaplan, M.D.
Kimberly A. Leite-Morris, B.S.

Cellular Biology of the Neuron

The human brain contains approximately 100 billion neurons that are interconnected within complex circuits via multiple synaptic connections. The essence of neural function is the signaling of, or information transfer by, an intracellular passage of information from one part of the cell to another and an intercellular passage of information between cells. This complex network through which neurons communicate allows the brain to sense changes in the environment, interpret the sensory stimuli, generate complex motor and behavioral responses, and store the information in the form of memories.

The nervous system contains two groups of cells: neuronal and glial cells. Neurons are electrically polarized cells that are specialized for the conduction of electrical impulses. Glial cells support neuronal function as they perform myelination, maintain the extracellular environment, generate inflammatory responses, and secrete trophic factors. These two groups include many subtypes of cells, each with different structure, function, and chemistry. In this section we describe the basic structure of neuronal and glial cells.

Neuronal cells have four distinct components: the soma, dendrites, axons, and presynaptic terminals. The soma, or cell body, may exist in a variety of shapes; it contains organelles for making ribonucleic acids and proteins, the same components that one would find in any other mammalian cell. The following cell structures are found within the

This work was supported by a Merit Review Grant from the Department of Veterans Affairs.

cytoplasm of neurons: the nucleus (contains the cell's genetic material), rough and smooth endoplasmic reticulum (sites of protein synthesis and transport), the Golgi apparatus (site of protein sorting and modification), mitochondria (sites of cellular oxidative metabolism), lysosomes (sites for degradation of cellular waste), and neurotubules and neurofilaments (important in cellular transport) (Brady et al. 1999; Raine 1999) (Figure 2–1).

Nucleic acids, deoxyribonucleic acid (DNA) and ribonucleic acid (RNA), and proteins are the essential building blocks of cells (see Figure 2–1). The information contained in the double-helical strands of DNA serves as a template for the transcription of DNA into RNA, called messenger RNA (mRNA). Information contained in mRNA is translated for protein synthesis. The entire process is known as *gene expression:*

DNA————TRANSCRIPTION————→mRNA————TRANSLATION————→PROTEIN

Each neuron contains thousands of genes and therefore can express thousands of different RNA messages, which can be further modified to form an enormous array of proteins during posttranslational processing. These protein molecules are of different shapes and sizes and have various functions; they are the elements that characterize neurons.

DNA is composed of a string of nucleotides, certain sequences of which represent genes. The four nucleotides that make up DNA are the purines adenine (A) and guanine (G) and the pyrimidines cytosine (C) and thymine (T). The nucleotides for RNA are the same (A, G, C) as those for DNA except for uracil (U), which substitutes for thymine. The nucleotides are joined together into strands by phosphate bonds. Two strands join together by base pairing of a purine and a pyrimidine, so that C is complementary to G and A is complementary to T (or to U in RNA), thus forming a double helix. DNA remains in the nucleus, and one strand is used as a template to produce a strand of mRNA that is released and carries the genetic message from the nucleus to the cytoplasm in a process termed *transcription*. The mRNA that results from this process is called a *transcript*. Each sequence of three nucleotides specifies one amino acid and forms the genetic code. There are 20 amino acids that can assemble into different proteins in a process called *translation*, which takes place in the cytoplasm. In neurons, polypeptides are synthesized in the rough endoplasmic reticulum and then transported to the Golgi complex, where posttranslational modifications occur. The resulting proteins are delivered to exact intracellular positions. In this way, genetic information is used to define the structure and function of neuronal proteins (Brady et al. 1999).

Two types of processes—the axon and the dendrites—originate from the cell bodies of neurons. With few exceptions, only one axon extends from the soma. The axon is a tubular process specialized for intracellular information transfer. It can convey information long distances by propagation of a brief electrical signal along its length, called an *action potential*. The axon originates from a funnel-shaped thickening of the cell body, called the *axon hillock*. It is here that the action potential initiates. Neurons give rise to multiple dendritic processes that are thicker, shorter, and more highly branched compared with axons. The branching of the dendrites resembles a tree (Kandel et al. 1990). As an organism develops, the numbers of and connections between axons and dendrites increase. The remodeling of these dendritic connections occurs through all stages of development and correlates with changes in neuronal functions. Postsynaptic processes on dendrites receive and integrate synaptic responses from multiple neuronal inputs (see Figure 2–1).

Messages are passed from neuron to neuron by being transmitted across the synapse, an apposition of the plasma membranes forming a presynaptic and a postsynaptic junction. An electrical impulse traveling down the axon, away from the cell body, is converted into a chemical signal at the synapse. Generally, the presynaptic terminal releases neurotransmitter from vesicular stores into the synaptic cleft, where it acts upon the postsynaptic process membrane. At the postsynaptic membrane, the chemical signal may either be converted into an electrical signal or be transduced into an intracellular (chemical) signal.

Neurons are classified according to several different parameters, such as the number of axons and dendrites (neurites) that extend from the soma. If a cell has one neurite, it is unipolar; if it has two neurites, it is bipolar; and if it has three or more neurites, it is considered multipolar. Neurons may also be classified by their shape, location, or function. Pyramidal cells (pyramidal in shape) and stellate cells (starlike in shape) are located in the cerebral cortex. Neurons that deliver signals from sensory receptors at external surfaces of the body (e.g., mechanoreceptors in the skin) to the central nervous system (CNS) are called *primary sensory* neurons. Neurons that innervate muscles are called *motor* neurons; those forming connections with other neurons are called *interneurons*. Neurons with long axons extending from one area of the brain to another are called *Golgi Type I* or *projection* neurons (e.g., pyramidal cells). Alternatively, nerve cells with short axons not extending beyond the cell body are called *Golgi Type II* or *local circuit* neurons (e.g., stellate cells). Neurons also may be classified on the basis of their neurotransmitter content; for example, those that release dopamine are referred to as *dopaminergic* cells.

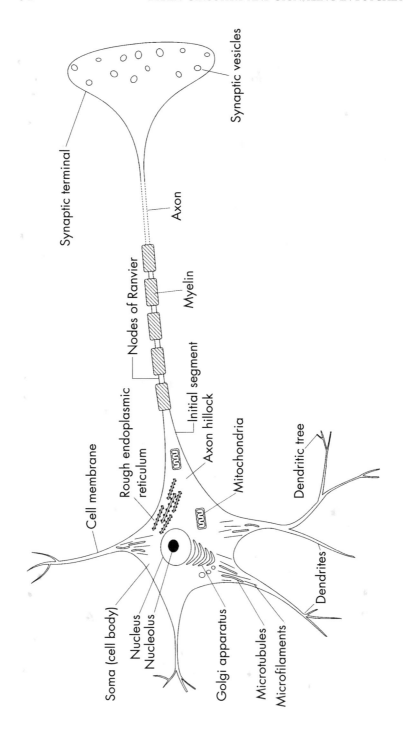

Figure 2-1. *The neuron has four distinct regions: the cell body (soma), an axon, dendrites, and a presynaptic terminal. The soma contains the nucleus and the cytoplasmic organelles (including mitochondria, rough endoplasmic reticulum containing ribosomes, and the Golgi apparatus). The Golgi apparatus packages newly synthesized proteins from the ribosomes into secretory organelles for transport out of the cell. The neuron is rich in microtubules and microfilaments that may provide support for axons and dendrites and assist in the transport of organelles. The axon has fine branches at its end called presynaptic terminals (shown enlarged in this figure), which release neurotransmitters from vesicles to other neurons. Transmitter molecules are stored in the synaptic vesicles located at the terminal; during depolarization, the contents of the vesicles are deposited into the synaptic cleft. The terminals make contact with other neurons that receive the signal; thus, these neurons are called the postsynaptic cells.*

The brain contains glial cells, which are not involved in information processing but which contribute to the function of the brain by insulating, supporting, and nourishing neurons. *Astrocytes* are the most abundant type of glial cell and are interposed between neurons, surrounding the synaptic junction. Unique proteins of the astrocytes can remove neurotransmitters from the synapse, limiting their dispersion beyond the synaptic cleft. Astrocytes also possess neurotransmitter receptors that can elicit electrical and biochemical signals inside the glial cell. Myelinating glia consist of two other types of glial cell: in the CNS, oligo-dendrocytes myelinate several axons, and in peripheral nerves, Schwann cells myelinate single axons. These cells insulate axons by wrapping them with layers of membrane (referred to as *myelin*); the entire covering is called the *myelin sheath.* The interruptions along this sheath where the axon is exposed are called the *nodes of Ranvier.* Two other types of cells also exist in the brain: ependymal cells, which line the ventricles, and microglia, which function as phagocytes to remove cellular debris (Raine 1999).

Nerve Conductance and Synaptic Transmission

Neurons receive and integrate multiple synaptic inputs and then generate electrical activity in their cell bodies, axons, and dendrites. To understand the process of neuronal conduction, it is first necessary to understand the physiology of the neuron at rest. Neuronal cells at rest are electrically polarized due to a separation of ionic charges between the relatively positive extracellular and relatively negative intracellular environments. This electrical potential is maintained by a high extracellular concentration of sodium, calcium, and chloride along with high intracellular concentrations of potassium. Separation of charges results in an electrical potential that is actively maintained by a selectively permeable lipid membrane and by ion channels. Ion channels are proteins with pores that selectively allow the flow of ions down a concentration gradient. A neuron's *equilibrium potential* is determined by the balance of thermodynamic and electrostatic forces established by ionic concentration gradients and voltage differences, respectively, with no net flow of ions. At this potential, an ion is as likely to move through an ion channel following a concentration gradient as it is to move in the opposite direction due to electrostatic forces. Neurons maintain ion concentration gradients through active transport pumps, such as the sodium-potassium pump. This pump maintains a relatively negative membrane potential in neurons by moving sodium out of and potassium into cells using energy from adenosine triphosphate (ATP) molecules (McCormick 1999).

Voltage-gated sodium, calcium, and potassium channels contribute to the generation of electrical signals in neurons through action potentials. An increase in membrane potential or depolarization enhances the cell's ability to conduct a signal along the axon. Upon reaching the threshold potential, this brief depolarization event (<1 millisecond) results in an action potential. The initial phase of this potential arises via a rapid increase in sodium permeability through voltage-sensitive sodium channels. Next, the repolarization phase of the action potential is produced via potassium channels, which permit outward potassium flux. The action potential is restored to the resting potential after a *hyperpolarization* or increase in charge separation occurs. Electrical excitation of adjoining ion channels along the axon results in the continuation of the action potential along the length of the axon. Such action potentials are able to travel over long distances without a lessening of the signal (Catterall 1995).

A *slow potential* is a localized membrane potential that develops over longer time periods (milliseconds to minutes) and can result in either depolarizations or hyperpolarizations. These potentials often arise out of neurotransmitter-receptor interactions that result in the opening of a different type of ion channel, a *ligand-gated* ion channel. Such potentials reflect the intensity of the stimulus, are spatially and temporally summed within a cell, and travel only short distances. Neurotransmitter receptors carry out their functions via either intracellular biochemical cascades (metabotropic receptors; Figures 2–2 and 2–3) or ion channels (ionophoric receptors; Figure 2–4). Activation of some types of receptors (e.g., ionotropic glutamate receptors) results in an increase in membrane permeability to positively charged ions such as sodium or calcium, which produces a depolarizing slow potential or an excitatory postsynaptic potential (EPSP). With other types of receptors, such as γ-aminobutyric acid (GABA) receptors, stimulation increases permeability of negatively charged ions (e.g., chloride), producing hyperpolarization of the membrane or an inhibitory postsynaptic potential (IPSP). Finally, stimulation of postsynaptic metabotropic receptors activates biochemical cascades that have downstream effects on ion channels (e.g., potassium or calcium efflux). In any given postsynaptic cell, numerous synaptic inputs are integrated from these slow potentials. Whether or not an action potential is generated in a given cell depends on the membrane properties of the cell and the intensity and location of synaptic inputs of these EPSPs and IPSPs (Kandel et al. 1990).

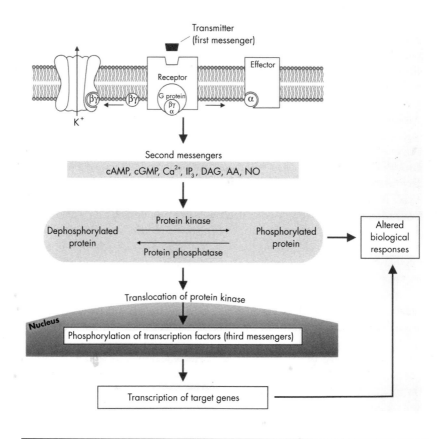

Figure 2–2. *Metabotropic receptors activate different effector enzymes and ion channels, resulting in an intracellular cascade of events. A neurotransmitter or first messenger binds to a cell surface coupled to the effector enzymes or channels via G proteins. Activation of G protein–coupled receptors results in the exchange of guanosine 5′-triphosphate (GTP) for guanosine 5′-diphosphate (GDP) on the α subunit of the G protein α, β, and γ complex. Free α subunits, which are bound to GTP, stimulate or inhibit the effectors. Free β-γ subunits directly activate a potassium (K$^+$) ion channel, thereby initiating the opening of the channel. An enzymatic function within the G protein hydrolyzes GTP and promotes the reassociation of α and β-γ subunits. Second messengers activate protein kinases that phosphorylate many protein components, such as metabotropic receptors, ion channels, and transcription factors. Phosphorylation of certain transcription factors promotes their binding to regulatory regions of various target genes and increases their rate of transcription. cAMP = cyclic adenosine 3′,5′-monophosphate; cGMP = cyclic guanosine monophosphate; Ca^{2+} = calcium; IP$_3$ = inositol 1,4,5-triphosphate; DAG = diacylglycerol; AA = arachidonic acid; NO = nitric oxide.*

The arrival of an action potential at the end of an axon results in chemical transmission across the synapse. Depolarization in the presynaptic neuron opens voltage-sensitive calcium channels in the nerve terminal, creating calcium flux into the cell. Calcium influx produces fusion of neurotransmitter-containing vesicles with the synaptic plasma membrane in a process known as *exocytosis*. This results in rapid release of neurotransmitters into the synapse and regeneration of new synaptic vesicles for storage. Neurotransmitters diffuse across the synapse, and signaling is resumed in the postsynaptic neuron by transmitter-induced activation of receptors. Termination of neurotransmitter actions occurs via diffusion of the neurotransmitter away from the binding site of the receptor, followed by its active reuptake into the presynaptic terminal or adjacent glial cell, or by its metabolism via enzymes. Neurotransmitters transduce their signals to the postsynaptic cell via receptors coupled either to ion channels or to enzyme effector systems that directly or indirectly produce electrical potential changes (De Camilli and Takei 1996; Holz and Fisher 1999).

Role of Signal Transduction in Synaptic Transmission

[handwritten annotation: To convert input energy of one form to output energy of another form]

Intracellular signaling pathways connect the neuronal cell surface to the nucleus through a process known as *signal transduction*. Signaling is initiated by the interaction of extracellular signals, or first messengers (e.g., neurotransmitters or drugs), with membrane receptors on the neuronal cell surface. Neurotransmitter receptors are membrane-spanning proteins that recognize and bind neurotransmitters as ligands and activate either ion channels or intracellular second-messenger systems via effector enzymes. There are several types of neurotransmitter receptor–mediated signals in brain cells: ligand-gated ion channels, G protein–coupled receptors, receptors with intrinsic kinase activity, and intracellular receptors. Neurotransmitter activation of ligand-gated ion channels results in increased permeability of these channels and produces fast synaptic actions (see Figure 2–4). G protein–coupled receptors do not mediate their intracellular effects directly but do so instead via signal-transducing G proteins. These receptors are coupled either to ion channels or to second-messenger systems that act upon intracellular targets (see Figures 2–2 and 2–3). A receptor with intrinsic kinase activity, such as tyrosine kinase, may bind to growth factor, resulting in the autophosphorylation of tyrosine residues on the receptors. Such effects produce clustering of effector proteins around the growth factor–recep-

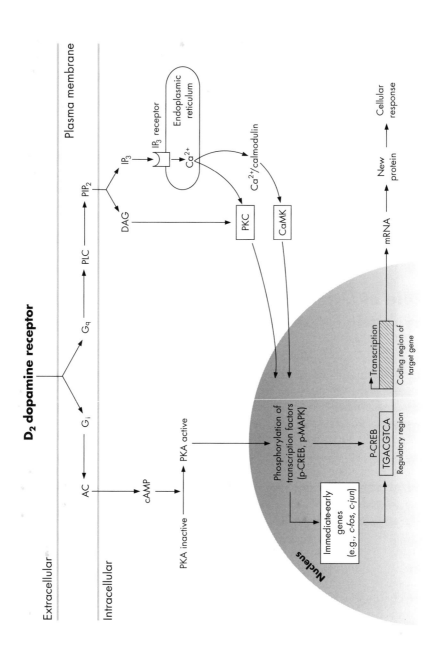

Figure 2–3. *Dopamine receptor signaling via the phosphatidylinositide and cyclic adenosine 3',5'-monophosphate (cAMP) pathway. D_2 dopamine receptor activation produces inhibition of the effector enzyme adenylyl cyclase (AC) or activation of phospholipase C (PLC) via coupling to G proteins G_i and G_q, respectively. With AC inhibition, cAMP levels are reduced and the regulatory protein kinase A (PKA) subunits are free to combine with the catalytic subunits, producing the inactive form of the enzyme. D_2 receptor activation also stimulates the hydrolysis of phosphatidylinositol 4,5-bis-phosphate (PIP_2) and the formation of two second messengers: diacylglycerol (DAG) and inositol 1,4,5-triphosphate (IP_3). IP_3 binds to its receptor on the endoplasmic reticulum and stimulates the release of calcium, resulting in activation of protein kinase C (PKC) and Ca^{2+}/calmodulin-dependent protein kinase (CaMK). D_2 antagonist drugs, such as antipsychotics, regulate the activity of PKC, PKA, and CaMK, which in turn regulate the phosphorylation of transcription factor CREB. Antipsychotics may alter neuronal responses by regulating CREB phosphorylation via CRE-mediated inducible expression of target genes. Ca^{2+} = calcium; CREB = cAMP response element binding; CRE = cAMP response element; MAPK = mitogen-activated protein kinase.*

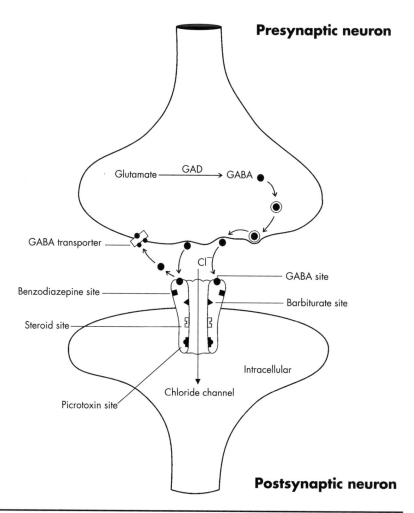

Figure 2–4. *The γ-aminobutyric acid A (GABA_A) receptor (shown enlarged in the postsynaptic neuron) is the primary ionotropic receptor involved in fast inhibitory synaptic transmission in the brain. The GABA_A receptor has a complex pharmacology in that it contains five binding domains that modulate its response to GABA stimulation. The binding areas are located at or within the ion channel and include sites for GABA, barbiturates, benzodiazepines, anesthetics, steroids, and picrotoxin. GABA is formed presynaptically by the enzyme glutamic acid decarboxylase (GAD), packaged into synaptic vesicles, and released into the synaptic cleft. The neurotransmitter diffuses across the cleft and binds to target postsynaptic receptors. A bidirectional transport system allows for the reutilization of GABA. The activation of GABA_A receptors hyperpolarizes neuronal cells and therefore inhibits their firing. Cl⁻ = chloride.*

tor complex, resulting in production of second messengers. Intracellular receptors are proteins that bind to peptides or steroid hormones, such as cortisol or gonadal steroids, and then diffuse to the nucleus, where they regulate gene transcription (Holz and Fisher 1999).

G proteins, or guanine nucleotide-binding proteins, are signaling proteins that link the external receptor with the internal effector response (see Figure 2–2). Dopaminergic, serotonergic, cholinergic, adenosinergic, and adrenergic receptors all use G protein–mediated signaling. As a ligand binds to its receptors, a conformational change occurs in the activated receptor complex and a cytoplasmic domain of the receptor makes contact with the G proteins. G proteins are composed of three polypeptide subunits, α, β, and γ; guanosine diphosphate (GDP) is bound to the α subunit. Receptor activation catalyzes the exchange of guanosine triphosphate (GTP) for GDP on the α subunit, producing its dissociation from the β and γ subunits. Free α and β-γ subunits are able to regulate multiple effector enzymes and ion channels, such as adenylyl cyclase, phospholipase, potassium, and calcium channels. An enzymatic function within the G protein (guanosine triphosphatase [GTPase] activity) hydrolyzes GTP to GDP and promotes the reassociation of α and β-γ subunits (Neer 1995).

An important function of G proteins is their ability to produce intracellular signal amplification. Each neurotransmitter receptor can activate multiple G proteins, each G protein can activate multiple effectors, and each effector can synthesize large numbers of intracellular second messengers. Each second messenger is capable of activating a protein kinase enzyme that regulates the function of many cellular signaling elements via phosphorylation. In this manner, G proteins provide both branching and integration of signals. Cross-talk between different signaling cascades occurs through both G proteins and second messengers that function in multiple cascades. Because G proteins integrate signaling from various receptors, ion channels, and effectors, they represent an important site for the coordination and integration of neuronal output. G proteins provide a range of temporal signals by activating both rapid (ion channel) and slower (second messenger) forms of signaling (Schulman and Hyman 1999).

Second Messenger–Protein Kinase Systems

The transduction of the extracellular signal to the intracellular portion of the neuron triggers an amplification of the signal via production of large numbers of low-molecular-weight second messengers (e.g., cyclic adenosine 3',5'-monophosphate [cAMP]). Second messengers act on intracellular targets, such as protein kinases, that phosphorylate various target proteins. *Protein kinases* are enzymes that transfer phosphate groups from ATP to serine, threonine, and tyrosine amino-acid residues on proteins, thereby altering their function. Protein kinases are activated by second messengers such as cAMP, calcium/calmodulin, and diacylglycerol. *Protein phosphatases* are intracellular proteins that hydrolyze phosphoryl groups from these same phosphorylated amino acids on target proteins (see Figure 2–2). Protein kinases and phosphatases regulate the state of phosphorylation of proteins, providing opportunities for signal coordination and amplification. Synaptic responsivity and neuronal excitability are modulated by the balance of phosphorylated and de-phosphorylated forms of proteins, such as ion channels, synaptic vesicle proteins, receptors, structural proteins, and enzymes. Phosphorylation of these proteins alters the processes of neurotransmitter synthesis and release and of neuronal growth (Girault and Greengard 1999; Schulman and Hyman 1999).

The cAMP pathway is one important example of a second messenger–induced protein kinase cascade (see Figure 2–3). This cascade is mediated by the enzyme *adenylyl cyclase*, which synthesizes cAMP from ATP, and certain phosphodiesterases enzymatically degrade cAMP. Multiple isoforms of adenylyl cyclase (types I–VIII) exist in the brain and differ in their distribution and regulation. Each isoform of this enzyme is regulated by α or β-γ subunits of G proteins, by calcium/calmodulin, or by phosphorylation. cAMP has many intracellular functions, including activation of a specific protein kinase, cAMP-dependent protein kinase (PKA), that phosphorylates structural and signaling proteins. PKA is a protein with two regulatory and two catalytic subunits that are inactive until stimulated. The binding of cAMP to regulatory subunits allows the catalytic subunits to dissociate and to phosphorylate cytoplasmic and nuclear substrate proteins (Girault and Greengard 1999).

The free catalytic subunits of PKA phosphorylate proteins and play a role in gene transcription. PKA catalytic subunits translocate to neuronal nuclei, where they can promote transcription of cAMP-responsive genes by phosphorylating a transcription factor known as *cAMP response element binding (CREB) protein*. Phosphorylation of the serine moiety at position 133 (Ser[133]) of the CREB protein promotes the binding of this protein (phosphoCREB) to a cAMP-responsive element (CRE), or protein-DNA binding region, in the promoter of various genes. PhosphoCREB binding to CREs in the promoter region of several genes increases their rate of transcription. CREB-induced changes in gene transcription may enhance synaptic efficacy, thus providing the cellular basis for the plasticity-induced memory formation (Girault and Greengard 1999; Mochly-Rosen 1995).

Another important second-messenger system is derived from the structure of neuronal phospholipid membranes (see Figure 2–3). The *phosphatidylinositide pathway* involves neurotransmitter receptor–coupled hydrolysis of membrane phospholipids (e.g., phosphatidylinositol 4,5-bis-phosphate, or PIP_2) by the enzyme phospholipase C (PLC). PLC produces a variety of phosphoinositide second messengers, such as inositol 1,4,5-triphosphate (IP_3) and diacylglycerol (DAG). These inositol phosphates liberate calcium from endoplasmic reticulum, and both DAG and calcium activate protein kinase C (PKC). PKC is another in the family of serine/threonine kinases, but it is associated with phosphatidylinositide and calcium signaling. Like other protein kinases, PKC phosphorylates important proteins involved in neurotransmitter release, gene expression, ion channel function, and receptor signaling. IP_3 is inactivated by phosphatases to inositol, and this by-product is incorporated back into the cellular membrane. Chronic treatment with lithium reduces inositol as its major mechanism of action and dampens neurotransmitter-mediated activation of this signaling pathway (Manji et al. 1995).

Calcium/calmodulin signaling is another important second-messenger system (see Figure 2–3). Calcium concentrations in extracellular spaces are high relative to those in the intracellular milieu. Intracellular calcium concentrations are rapidly increased by activation of neurotransmitter-gated calcium channels and voltage-gated channels and by mobilization of intracellular calcium stores. Many G protein–coupled receptors initiate calcium signaling through PLC, and this produces second-messenger inositol phosphates. Inositol phosphates bind to intracellular receptors, resulting in release from intracellular calcium stores in the endoplasmic reticulum. The major intracellular mediator of calcium's actions is the protein *calmodulin.* Calcium binds to sites on calmodulin, thereby enhancing calmodulin's affinity for other enzymes, such as protein kinases, adenylyl cyclase, and phosphodiesterase. Finally, calcium activates a family of calcium/calmodulin-dependent protein kinases (CaM kinases). CaM kinases phosphorylate a host of proteins in the neuron, including enzymes (e.g., tyrosine hydroxylase), structural proteins, transcription factors, and receptors. CaM kinases and PKA also have been implicated in molecular mechanisms of memory (Clapham 1995; Schulman and Hyman 1999).

Second Messenger–Induced Gene Transcription and Synaptic Remodeling

Process of copying genetic info from DNA in chromosomes to ribosomes in cytoplasm into proteins

Because proteins such as receptors and enzymes are degraded continually in neurons, new protein synthesis is a ongoing requirement. Transcription and translation represent amplification processes in which a single gene produces thousands of mRNAs and a single mRNA is translated into hundreds of proteins. Certain portions of the genome contain encoding regions in which the sequence of nucleotides is translated into a precise arrangement of amino acids for a given protein. Control regions of the DNA determine which specific genes are to be expressed in a cell. Regulation of gene expression occurs via nuclear proteins, such as immediate-early gene products or other transcription factors, which bind to specific sequences of DNA. Immediate-early genes (e.g., *c-fos*) rapidly transcribe several types of nuclear DNA-binding proteins, such as Fos and Jun, in response to extracellular signals and/or neuronal depolarization (see Figure 2–3). The binding of nuclear proteins to DNA control sequences alters transcription of target genes. Inducible gene transcription can result in production of new cellular proteins and mediate long-term adaptive cellular changes and synaptic remodeling (Hyman and Nestler 1999).

Neural plasticity refers to stimulus-induced changes in synaptic strength, and this underlies complex processes such as learning, psychotherapeutic drug effects, and drug addiction. This adaptation of the brain is shaped by both environmental (e.g., experiences and drug treatments) and endogenous (e.g., neurotransmitter and hormonal) factors. Alteration in synaptic connections results from changes in synaptic protein function (via phosphorylation) or protein levels (via inducible processes of transcription). Stimulus-induced changes in gene transcription can result in production of new proteins and rearrangement of synaptic connections that mediate long-term behavioral changes. In the developing brain, axons establish connections with target neurons to create neural circuits. Once the connections are established, the addition or subtraction of synapses can modify these circuits. Neuronal plasticity underlies the organism's ability to change its behavior or to learn by reshaping synaptic connections. *Long-term potentiation* (LTP) is an example of transcription-induced neuronal plasticity that results in enhanced synaptic connectivity and that may represent the cellular basis for memory (Hyman and Nestler 1999).

Role of Specific Neurotransmitters and Neuromodulators in Synaptic Transmission

Multiple neurotransmitter substances are expressed by individual neurons. Stimulation of a neuron produces the release of neurotransmitters from presynaptic vesicles and diffusion of these substances to specific binding sites on receptors. At a given moment, a neuron is influenced by the summation of thousands of synaptic events that are regulated by neurotransmitter-mediated signal transduction via ion channels and second messengers. The functional response in the postsynaptic neuron depends on the temporal and spatial summation of these neurotransmitter receptor potentials. An understanding of the major neurotransmitter signaling pathways is critically important in comprehending the basis of neuropsychiatric conditions and their treatments.

Dopamine

Dopaminergic signaling plays a critical role in psychiatric conditions such as schizophrenia and drug addiction (see Chapters 3 and 4 in this volume). The midbrain has several major dopaminergic neuronal pathways that synthesize, store, and release dopamine, including the nigrostriatal (A9) and mesocorticolimbic (A10) pathways. In the nigrostriatal pathway, dopamine-containing cell bodies located in the substantia nigra project to the dorsal striatum or to the caudate and putamen. The mesocorticolimbic pathway originates from neurons in the ventral tegmental area and terminates in two forebrain regions: the ventral striatum (including the nucleus accumbens and olfactory tubercle) and the cortex (including the prefrontal, anterior cingulate, and entorhinal cortices). There are also dopamine-containing cell bodies in the hypothalamus that send projections to the pituitary and regulate prolactin function. The rate and pattern of dopaminergic neuronal firing correlate with the amount of dopamine released (Deutch and Roth 1999).

All catecholamines (dopamine, norepinephrine, epinephrine) are synthesized in the CNS from the amino acid tyrosine. Tyrosine, like most amino acids, cannot cross the blood-brain barrier by passive diffusion; instead, it is taken up into the brain by active transport. In the biosynthesis of all catecholamines, the conversion of tyrosine to L-dopa is catalyzed by tyrosine hydroxylase, the rate-limiting enzyme in catecholamine synthesis. L-dopa is then converted to dopamine by the enzyme DOPA decarboxylase. Dopamine is taken up into storage vesicles and released at nerve terminals via a calcium-dependent mechanism. The action of dopamine at the synapse is terminated via reuptake into the presynaptic terminal by transporter proteins. Intraneuronal dopamine either is transported into vesicles by the vesicular monoamine transporter or is metabolized to dihydroxyphenylacetic acid (DOPAC) by the enzyme monoamine oxidase (MAO). Extraneuronal dopamine is converted to homovanillic acid (HVA) via the actions of catechol-*O*-

methyltransferase (COMT). Thus, the functional activity of dopaminergic neurons can be evaluated by assessing the accumulation of HVA in the brain or cerebrospinal fluid (Boulton and Eisenhofer 1998; Deutch and Roth 1999).

There are six known subtypes of dopamine receptors (D_1, D_{2L}, D_{2S}, D_3, D_4, and D_5), which are divided into two major groups: D_1-like (D_1 and D_5) and D_2-like (D_2, D_3, and D_4) (Table 2–1). Dopamine receptors belong to a family of G protein–coupled receptors. The amino acid sequence of each of these receptor subtypes has a characteristic seven-membrane-spanning region. D_1 and D_5 dopamine receptors are coupled to a stimulatory G protein (G_s) that activates adenylyl cyclase. D_2 receptors are coupled to an inhibitory G protein (G_i) that inhibits adenylyl cyclase. Therefore, D_2 receptors can regulate cAMP levels and downstream PKA. In some cell types, D_2 dopamine receptors stimulate phosphoinositol hydrolysis via phospholipase C activation. By enhancing the production of inositol triphosphate, D_2 receptors increase intracellular calcium levels and regulate downstream PKC (see Figure 2–3). D_2 receptors are also able to inhibit calcium currents and regulate potassium channels. D_1 receptors are expressed at the highest concentrations of all dopamine receptors and are found in the striatum, nucleus accumbens and other limbic regions, hypothalamus, and thalamus. D_5 receptors are found predominantly in the hippocampus and thalamus and are expressed at much lower concentrations. D_2 dopamine receptors are expressed in the neurons of the striatum and nucleus accumbens and are found on dopaminergic neurons in the ventral tegmental area, where they function as autoreceptors. The D_3 receptor is distributed in limbic regions, with relatively low expression in the striatum. D_4 receptors are present in frontal cortical and limbic areas, with less expression in the striatum (Jaber et al. 1996).

D_2 receptors are localized both on the cell body and on the terminals of dopaminergic neurons. They serve as inhibitory autoreceptors—their activation inhibits the rate of neuronal firing and reduces the release of dopamine at the nerve terminal. D_2 dopamine agonists inhibit and D_2 dopamine antagonists enhance the release of dopamine. The dopamine transporter is located at the dopamine nerve terminal, where it serves to inactivate and recycle dopamine from the synaptic cleft into the nerve terminal (Jaber et al. 1996). The clinical potency of antipsychotic agents closely correlates with their affinity for D_2 dopamine receptors. Because D_2 receptors are located in the striatum, their blockade is presumed to contribute to the extrapyramidal side effects of antipsychotic drugs. Because D_3 and D_4 dopamine receptors are found at relatively higher concentrations in the limbic system and cerebral cortex than in the striatum, selective D_3 and D_4 antagonists produce antipsy-

Table 2–1. *Neurotransmitter receptors and their effector mechanisms*

Neurotransmitter	Receptor subtype	Function[a]	Effector mechanism
Acetylcholine	Muscarinic:		
	$M_{1,3}$	GPL	↑ IP_3/DAG
	$M_{2,4}$	GPL	↓ cAMP, ↑ K^+
	M_5	?	?
	Nicotinic: multiple isoforms	IR	↑ Na^+, ↑ K^+, ↑ Ca^{2+}
Adenosine	A_1	GPL	↓ cAMP, ↑ K^+, ↓ Ca^{2+}, ↑ IP_3/DAG
	A_{2A}	GPL	↑ cAMP
	A_{2B}	GPL	↑ cAMP, ↑ IP_3/DAG
	A_3	GPL	↓ cAMP, ↑ IP_3/DAG
GABA	$GABA_A$ (multiple isoforms)	IR	Cl^-
	$GABA_B$	GPL	↓ cAMP, ↑ K^+, ↓ Ca^{2+}
Dopamine	D_1, D_5	GPL	↑ cAMP
	D_2 (two isoforms)	GPL	↓ cAMP, ↑ K^+, ↓ Ca^{2+}, ↑ IP_3/DAG
	D_3	GPL	↓ cAMP
	D_4	GPL	↓ cAMP, ↑ K^+
Glutamate/aspartate	AMPA: Glu_{1-4}	IR	↑ Na^+, ↑ K^+
	KA: Glu_{5-7} $KA_{1,2}$	IR	↑ Na^+, ↑ K^+
	NMDA: $NMDA_{1,2A-D}$	IR	↑ Na^+, ↑ K^+, ↑ Ca^{2+}
	$mGluR_{1,5}$	GPL	↑ IP_3/DAG, ↑ Ca^{2+}; $mGluR_1$: ↑ cAMP
	$mGluR_{2,3}$	GPL	↓ cAMP
	$mGluR_{4,6,7,8}$	GPL	↓ cAMP

Table 2–1. Neurotransmitter receptors and their effector mechanisms (continued)

Neurotransmitter	Receptor subtype	Function[a]	Effector mechanism
Norepinephrine	α_{1A-D}	GPL	$\uparrow IP_3/DAG$
	α_{2A-C}	GPL	$\downarrow cAMP, \uparrow K^+, \downarrow Ca^{2+}$
	β_{1-3}	GPL	$\uparrow cAMP$
Opioid peptides	Mu (μ)	GPL	$\downarrow cAMP, \uparrow K^+, \downarrow Ca^{2+}$
	Delta (δ)	GPL	$\downarrow cAMP, \uparrow K^+, \downarrow Ca^{2+}$
	Kappa (κ)	GPL	$\downarrow cAMP, \uparrow K^+, \downarrow Ca^{2+}$
Serotonin	$5\text{-}HT_{1A-F}$	GPL	$\downarrow cAMP, \uparrow K^+$
	$5\text{-}HT_{2A-C}$	GPL	$\uparrow IP_3/DAG; 5\text{-}HT_{2A}: \downarrow K^+$
	$5\text{-}HT_3$	IR	$\uparrow Na^+, \uparrow K^+$
	$5\text{-}HT_{4,6,7}$	GPL	$\uparrow cAMP$
	$5\text{-}HT_5$	GPL	$\downarrow cAMP$

Note. AC = adenylyl cyclase; AMPA = α-amino-3-hydroxy-5-methyl-4-isoxalone propionic acid; Ca = calcium; cAMP = cyclic adenosine 3′,5′-monophosphate; Cl = chloride; DAG = diacylglycerol; GABA = γ-aminobutyric acid; 5-HT = 5-hydroxytryptamine (serotonin); IP_3 = inositol 1,4,5-triphosphate; K = potassium; KA = kainate; mGluR = metabotropic glutamate receptor; Na = sodium; NMDA = *N*-methyl-D-aspartate.
[a]GPL = G protein–linked receptor; IR = ionotropic receptor.
Source. Adapted from Bloom FE: "Neurotransmission and the Central Nervous System," in *Goodman and Gilman's The Pharmacological Basis of Therapeutics*, 9th Edition. Edited by Hardman JG, Limbird LE. New York, McGraw-Hill, 1996, pp. 267–294. Copyright 1996, The McGraw-Hill Companies. Used with permission.

chotic effects with a low incidence of extrapyramidal side effects (Grace et al. 1997).

Norepinephrine (Noradrenaline)

Norepinephrine-containing neurons are organized into dorsal and ventral groups in the pons and medulla. The dorsal, or pontine, group of neurons is located in the locus coeruleus and is the major group of noradrenergic nerve cells in the mammalian brain. These neurons project *dorsal NE* widely to the cerebral cortex, limbic regions, thalamus, hippocampus, cerebellum, and spinal cord. The ventral group is located in the medulla *ventral* and projects to the hypothalamus, locus coeruleus, and spinal cord. This wide distribution permits norepinephrine to play a role in multiple brain functions, including stress and autonomic responses, attention, memory, and mood. Furthermore, norepinephrine plays a major role in pathophysiological conditions such as anxiety, depression, and addiction. In norepinephrine-containing neurons, dopamine is converted to norepinephrine within vesicles by the enzyme dopamine β-hydroxylase. A small set of neurons in the brain stem contain the enzyme phenylethanolamine-N-methyltransferase (PNMT), which further catalyzes norepinephrine to epinephrine (Kuhar et al. 1999).

Synaptic norepinephrine levels are primarily regulated by transporter proteins, which are found on presynaptic terminals. The norepinephrine transporter can be blocked by tricyclic antidepressants and by venlafaxine, a newer antidepressant medication. As is the case with dopamine, the presynaptic mitochondrial enzyme MAO (there are two forms, MAO-A and MAO-B) inactivates norepinephrine that is not stored in vesicles. Synaptic norepinephrine levels are enhanced by certain drugs, such as phenelzine and other inhibitors of MAO. Additionally, the enzyme COMT inactivates norepinephrine in extraneuronal tissues. Drugs that alter the synthesis, storage, release, reuptake, and enzymatic degradation of the catecholamine neurotransmitters, along with several direct noradrenergic agonists and antagonists, aid in the treatment of diseases such as Parkinson's disease and hypertension (Boulton and Eisenhofer 1998; Kuhar et al. 1999).

Five main types of adrenergic receptors have been cloned (α_1, α_2, β_1, β_2, and β_3), all of which are G protein–coupled receptors (see Table 2–1). The major adrenergic receptors in the brain are α_2 and β_1. The α_1 adrenoreceptor has variant forms A–D (α_{1A-D}), and the α_2 receptor has variant forms A–C (α_{1A-C}); each receptor subtype has different regional specificity and functional properties. The binding of agonists to the α_1-adrenergic receptor enhances phosphatidylinositol turnover and calcium signaling. Activation of α_2-adrenergic receptors inhibits adenylyl cyclase activity, whereas activation of β-adrenergic receptors stimulates this effector. The α_2-adrenergic receptors serve as autoreceptors; their activation serves to inhibit norepinephrine release. Clonidine is an adrenergic agonist that binds to autoreceptors to exert inhibitory actions on norepinephrine release and on firing of noradrenergic neurons. Therefore, clonidine has utility in the treatment of anxiety and opiate withdrawal (Waxman 1999).

Serotonin

Serotonin is a key neurotransmitter with important roles in normal behavioral processes such as arousal, feeding, aggression, pain, circadian rhythmicity, and neuroendocrine function. It also has a key role in psychopathological conditions such as depression, anxiety, and addiction. Although serotonin is found in only a small percentage (about 1%–2%) of the neurons in the brain, its effects are widespread. Clusters of serotonergic cell bodies are located along the midline of the brain stem, known as raphe nuclei, and their axonal projections are distributed throughout the CNS. The dorsal and median raphe nuclei send projections to diverse regions including the cortex, hippocampus, limbic structures, striatum, thalamus, midbrain, and hypothalamus. The caudal raphe nuclei provide descending projections to the spinal cord (Deutch and Roth 1999).

Serotonin (5-hydroxytryptamine, or 5-HT) is synthesized in the neuron from its precursor amino acid, tryptophan, which is derived from the diet via active transport in the gut. The transport of this primary substrate is in direct competition with transport of other neutral amino acids, including tyrosine and phenylalanine (aromatic amino acids), leucine, isoleucine, and valine (branched-chain amino acids). Therefore, tryptophan uptake is related not only to tryptophan blood levels but also to plasma concentrations of other neutral amino acids. Plasma tryptophan concentrations fluctuate accordingly, and this affects the rate of serotonin synthesis. The enzyme tryptophan hydroxylase (L-tryptophan-5-monooxygenase), which converts tryptophan to 5-hydroxytryptophan (5-HTP), is the rate-limiting enzyme in serotonin synthesis; it is expressed only in serotonergic neurons. 5-HTP is then catalyzed by the aromatic amino acid decarboxylase (AADC), giving rise to serotonin (5-HT). Tryptophan hydroxylase is activated upon its phosphorylation by calcium/calmodulin and PKA. Chronic drug treatment and stress can alter the amount of tryptophan hydroxylase available (Frazer and Hensler 1999).

Serotonin is stored in synaptic vesicles prior to its release into the synapse by calcium-dependent exocytosis. Release of serotonin is primarily regulated by presynaptic 5-HT$_{1A}$ autoreceptors. The primary mechanism of serotonin inactivation is reuptake into the nerve terminal by transporter proteins. These transporter proteins are the targets of many drugs, including antidepressants and psychostimulants. MAO inactivates serotonin as well as catecholamines not stored in vesicles, and COMT degrades these neurotransmitters at extraneuronal sites (Frazer and Hensler 1999).

There are three families of G protein–coupled metabotropic serotonin receptors: the 5-HT$_1$, the 5-HT$_2$, and the 5-HT$_{4-7}$ subtypes (see Table 2–1). The 5-HT$_1$ receptor family contains the 5-HT$_{1A}$, 5-HT$_{1B}$, 5-HT$_{1D}$, 5-HT$_{1E}$, and 5-HT$_{1F}$ receptors, all of which are negatively coupled to adenylyl cyclase; their stimulation inhibits cAMP production. Additionally, the 5-HT$_{1A}$ receptor is coupled to ligand-gated ion channels. The 5-HT$_{1C}$ and 5-HT$_2$ receptor (5-HT$_{2A}$, 5-HT$_{2B}$, 5-HT$_{2C}$) families regulate phosphoinositide pathways and phospholipase C. The 5-HT$_4$, 5-HT$_5$, 5-HT$_6$, 5-HT$_7$ receptor families are positively coupled to adenylyl cyclase activity. Furthermore, the 5-HT$_3$ receptor family is ionotropic and is permeable to sodium and potassium. These serotonin receptors differ in their localization, which also reflects their differing functions (Murphy et al. 1998).

5-HT$_2$ receptors are of great importance in schizophrenia and in the action of antipsychotic drugs. These receptors are found on serotonergic projections to midbrain neurons; their activation enhances nigrostriatal, mesolimbic, and mesocortical dopamine cell firing. Conversely, 5-HT$_2$ antagonist drugs enhance nigrostriatal, mesolimbic, and mesocortical dopamine cell firing. By activating prefrontal cortical neurons, 5-HT$_2$ antagonist drugs may produce cognition-enhancing effects. By activating nigrostriatal dopamine cells, 5-HT$_2$ antagonist drugs may reduce extrapyramidal side effects. Drugs that enhance serotonergic transmission, such as serotonin reuptake inhibitors, are efficacious as anxiolytic, antidepressant, analgesic, and antiaggression agents (Chiodo and Bunney 1983).

Acetylcholine

Acetylcholine is found in the brain at cholinergic synapses and at the neuromuscular junction in the periphery. Cholinergic neurons contain the synthetic enzyme for acetylcholine, choline acetyltransferase (ChAT), and the enzyme that degrades acetylcholine, acetylcholinesterase (AChE). Cholinergic neurons are found as both broad-projecting neurons and local interneurons. Cholinergic neurons located in the nucleus basalis, diagonal band, and septum project widely and innervate the cortex and hippocampus. Neurons from the pedunculopontine tegmental nucleus project to regions in the cortex and spinal cord (Sarter and Bruno 1997). Acetylcholine's importance in attention and memory functions has been demonstrated by abundant research, including neuropathological findings of cholinergic neuronal degeneration as an etiological factor in Alzheimer's disease. Furthermore, treatment of patients with Alzheimer's disease with AChE inhibitors slows the progression of cognitive deterioration.

Acetylcholine is synthesized in a single synthetic step by the enzyme ChAT, which transfers the acetyl group from acetyl coenzyme A to choline. Acetylcholine formation is limited by the intracellular concentration of choline, which is taken up from plasma sources by a transport system. Acetyl coenzyme A arises from a variety of sources, including pyruvate, a product of glucose metabolism. Acetylcholine is transported to axons after being synthesized in the soma. Synaptic acetylcholine is taken up by a transporter protein into storage vesicles in the presynaptic terminal. Following exocytosis, is degraded by AChE via hydrolysis, producing choline, which is then available for reuptake (Deutch and Roth 1999).

Acetylcholine's actions are mediated by two types of receptors: nicotinic and muscarinic cholinergic receptors (see Table 2–1). These receptors are named for the action of their selective agonists, muscarine and nicotine. Most muscarinic receptors are G protein–coupled metabotropic receptors, of which five subtypes have been cloned (M_1–M_5). Muscarinic receptor subtypes are differentially distributed in the brain and exhibit different functional properties. M_1, M_3, and M_5 muscarinic receptors are coupled to IP_3/DAG systems. M_2 and M_4 muscarinic receptors are negatively coupled to adenylyl cyclase and also to G proteins that regulate potassium and calcium conductance. The nicotinic receptor is a ligand-gated ion channel consisting of a pentamer composed of two α and one each of subunits β, δ, and γ. Binding of acetylcholine to nicotinic receptor sites results in the influx of sodium and calcium and the efflux of potassium through a nonselective cation channel within the receptor complex. Some muscarinic agonists have important cognition-enhancing properties; nicotinic agonists also have cognition-activating effects in addition to their psychomotor-stimulant and reinforcing effects (Waxman 1999).

Glutamate

The amino acids glutamate and aspartate have been established as major excitatory neurotransmitters in the mammalian CNS. Glutamate is critically important in processes such as learning and memory, al-though excessive release can produce neuronal damage. Unlike the neurotransmitters described thus far, glutamate has been shown to act on virtually every neuron in the brain. Classified as nonessential amino acids, glutamate and aspartate cannot cross the blood-brain barrier and are produced by local brain synthesis. The metabolic and synthetic enzymes for glutamate and aspartate are found in both glial and neuronal cell sources. Glutamate can be synthesized via several different pathways, although how each pathway contributes to this synthesis is yet unknown. Glutamate is formed from glucose and the transamination of α-ketoglutarate in nerve terminals. Some glutamate is formed directly from glutamine in these terminals. Glutamine is synthesized in glial cells and is transported to neurons that replenish glutamate and GABA in the nerve terminals via the enzyme glutaminase. Many cell types use this neurotransmitter, including cortical motor neurons, cortical neurons projecting to the basal ganglia, granule cells of the cerebellum, and pyramidal cells in the hippocampus. Neurotransmission of glutamate is terminated by the rapid reuptake of the neurotransmitter by a glutamate transporter into the presynaptic axon terminal or into glial cells. Glutamate is taken up into synaptic vesicles and either metabolized to glutamine in glial cells or released again (Dingledine and McBain 1999).

There are three classes each of ionotropic and metabotropic glutamate receptors (see Table 2–1). One of the three ligand-gated channel receptors is the N-methyl-D-aspartate (NMDA) receptor, which functions as a voltage-dependent cation channel permitting the entrance of both sodium and calcium. The NMDA receptor has six known binding sites that regulate the probability of channel opening: glutamate, glycine, polyamine, magnesium, zinc, and hydrogen sites. NMDA, glutamate and aspartate are all agonists for the glutamate binding site. The NMDA receptor requires the binding of two different agonists—glutamate and glycine—for receptor activation. When glycine binds to the NMDA receptor, its conformation is altered and glutamate can then activate the channel. Occupancy of the other four binding sites modifies the opening of the ion channel. Even with glutamate and glycine binding to the NMDA receptor, the presence of magnesium at a site in the channel pore prevents ion passage. On the postsynaptic cell, the membrane must depolarize to remove NMDA receptor channel blockade by magnesium, after which the receptor will allow the passage of sodium and calcium (Dingledine and McBain 1999).

NMDA receptors have important roles in the development of synaptic plasticity via the induction of LTP. As discussed earlier, LTP is a phenomenon in which brief electrical stimulation produces long-lasting increases of postsynaptic responses. In LTP, calcium influx occurs via NMDA receptor channels only when synaptic input is sufficient to depolarize postsynaptic membranes and relieve magnesium blockade of these channels. Thus, LTP is an input-dependent phenomenon that involves NMDA receptor signaling. NMDA agonists and antagonists appear to have important roles both in cognition and in neuropsychiatric disorders such as stroke, epilepsy, schizophrenia, and drug addiction (Malenka and Nicoll 1999).

The other two ionotropic glutamate receptors are termed non-NMDA receptors and include α-amino-3-hydroxy-5-methyl-4-isoxalone propionic acid (AMPA) receptors and kainate receptors (see Table 2–1). Activation of kainate and AMPA receptors produces fast excitatory neurotransmission in the CNS via sodium channels. These receptors are often colocalized with NMDA receptors and are desensitized after receptor activation. Metabotropic glutamate receptors (mGluR) are classified into three groups based on their sequence homology and associated second-messenger systems. Group I receptors are coupled to phosphoinositide-specific phospholipase C and regulate intracellular calcium. Group II and III metabotropic receptors are coupled to adenylyl cyclase by a G protein; they regulate neurotransmitter release and are implicated in postsynaptic plasticity (Dingledine and McBain 1999).

GABA

GABA, the major inhibitory neurotransmitter in the mammalian CNS, is found both in local interneurons and in certain projection neurons. GABA is an amino acid derived from glucose metabolism in GABAergic neurons, where it is synthesized from glutamate by the enzyme glutamic acid decarboxylase (GAD) (see Figure 2–4). GAD is expressed only in neurons that synthesize and release GABA; thus, it provides an excellent marker of GABAergic neurons. The removal of synaptic GABA occurs either through degradation by GABA-transaminase in glial cells or through uptake at the nerve terminal by GABA transporters. Thirty percent of synapses use GABA, and its concentration in the brain is several orders of magnitude higher than the concentration of most other neurotransmitters. Depolarization of GABAergic neurons produces GABA release into the synaptic cleft, where the activation of postsynaptic receptors mediates its cellular actions (Deutch and Roth 1999).

GABA mediates its cellular effects by activating $GABA_A$, $GABA_B$, and $GABA_C$ receptor subtypes. The $GABA_A$ receptor is a ligand-gated ion (chloride) channel, whereas the $GABA_B$ receptor is a G protein–

coupled receptor. GABA$_A$ receptors contain heterogeneous subunits made up of five principal polypeptides: α, β, δ, ε, and γ. Different isoforms of GABA$_A$ receptors are found in nature, based on polypeptide subunit combinations, and each has its own unique pharmacological properties. GABA$_A$ receptors are allosterically modulated at five different recognition sites: the GABA, benzodiazepine, barbiturate, convulsant drug (picrotoxin), and steroid sites (see Figure 2–4). These sites modulate receptor responses to GABA activation. The binding of GABA to its recognition site directly opens chloride ion channels and results in cellular hyperpolarization. Benzodiazepine drugs (e.g., diazepam and other agonists) bind to their own recognition site, and this increases the frequency of channel opening in response to GABA. The binding of anesthetics, barbiturates, and alcohol to recognition sites on the channel complex enhances GABA-mediated chloride flux. GABA$_A$ receptor modulators, such as benzodiazepines, produce sedating, anxiolytic, reinforcing, and anticonvulsant effects (Mehta and Ticku 1999).

GABA$_B$ receptors are G protein–coupled receptors that are linked to various effectors, including adenylyl cyclase, potassium channels, and voltage-dependent calcium channels. Postsynaptic GABA$_B$ receptors activate inwardly rectifying potassium channels that produce sustained inhibitory postsynaptic potentials (IPSPs). Through their coupling with G$_i$ subunits, GABA$_B$ receptors inhibit adenylyl cyclase activity and reduce cAMP levels. Also, presynaptic GABA$_B$ receptor activation inhibits calcium conductance, and this results in reduced neurotransmitter release. There are two different subtypes of cloned GABA$_B$ receptors; full activity of the receptor appears to require the dimerization of both subunits. Treatment with GABA$_B$ receptor agonists produces muscle-relaxing and analgesic effects and inhibits aspects of drug addiction and craving. In most brain regions, GABA$_A$ receptors are present at higher density than GABA$_B$ receptors, and these latter receptors are found at the highest levels in the thalamus, cerebellum, cortex, and spinal cord. The GABA$_C$ receptor is composed of multiple ρ peptide subunits and is insensitive to GABA$_A$ agonists (e.g., muscimol) and GABA$_B$ agonists (e.g., baclofen) (Bowery and Enna 2000).

Adenosine

Adenosine is a neuromodulator produced mainly by the breakdown of extracellular nucleotides. During periods of increased metabolic activity and ischemia, greater levels of neuroprotective adenosine are created. Therefore, extracellular adenosine levels provide information about the metabolic state of cells. Extracellular adenosine is produced from ATP by a cascade of membrane-bound ectonucleotidases. ATP is released from cells during periods of heightened neuronal activity; its metabolite adenosine plays a neuroprotective role by inhibiting neuronal firing, presynaptic neurotransmitter release, and synaptic transmission. Adenosine levels are regulated by a bidirectional nucleoside transporter. Adenosine is metabolized by phosphorylation via adenosine kinase or by deamination by via adenosine deaminase. Extracellular adenosine acts at pre- and postsynaptic receptor sites. Adenosine binds to four high-affinity forms of G protein–coupled receptors: adenosine A_1, A_{2A}, A_{2B}, and A_3 subtypes (see Table 2–1). Adenosine A_1 and A_2 receptors are coupled to the enzyme adenylyl cyclase via G protein subtypes G_i and G_s, respectively. These adenosine receptors are also coupled to potassium and calcium channels and to the phosphatidylinositol system. Adenosine A_3 receptors are positively coupled to the phosphatidylinositol system. Adenosine A_1 receptors can be found presynaptically and regulate the release of neurotransmitters (e.g., dopamine, GABA, glutamate, norepinephrine) throughout the brain.

Adenosine A_{2A} receptors are collocated with D_2 dopamine receptors in striatopallidal neurons, and adenosine A_1 receptors are collocated with D_1 dopamine receptors in striatonigral neurons; each type of adenosine receptor inhibits the function of its colocalized dopamine receptor. Therefore, adenosine antagonists such as caffeine mediate their motor-stimulant effects by enhancing dopaminergic transmission in striatum (Ferre 1997; Meghji 1991). Adenosine agonists are known for their motor-suppressant, hypnotic, and anxiolytic effects and for their inhibition of actions of drugs of abuse. Adenosine A_{2A} and A_1 agonists inhibit the expression of drug (Kaplan et al. 1999a) and alcohol dependence (Kaplan and Sears 1996).

Neuropeptides

Neuropeptides are often released at synapses with neurotransmitters. Neuropeptides differ from neurotransmitters in that they are found at lower concentrations and are derived from large inactive precursor molecules synthesized in the soma. These neuropeptide precursors are transported down the axon while they are being cleaved and processed, and the peptides are degraded after synaptic release. Precursor peptides can be processed differently in different neurons, producing a diversity of related active peptides. For example, endogenous opioids are produced through enzymatic processing of the precursor neuropeptides proopiomelanocortin, proenkephalin, and prodynorphin, each of which has a unique anatomic distribution. Each precursor is broken down to different peptides with unique pharmacological effects and localizations.

Neuropeptides can act at multiple sites, including pre- and post-synaptic receptor sites, or even on cells farther away from their site of release. Peptides can exert endocrine effects by traveling in the blood circulation as releasing factors (e.g., corticotropin-releasing factor [CRF]) traveling from the hypothalamus to the pituitary or as pituitary hormones (e.g., adrenocorticotropic hormone [ACTH]) traveling to peripheral organs (e.g., adrenal cortex). Peptide release requires calcium influx. The quantity of release is proportional to neuronal firing. Most peptide-binding sites are G protein–coupled receptors that activate either ion channels or enzyme effectors. Peptides and neurotransmitters can produce similar physiological effects; however, these effects occur on different time scales (Mains and Eipper 1999).

Signaling Mechanisms of Psychotropic Drugs: The Example of Antipsychotics

Many psychoactive drugs alter neuronal signaling by functioning as endogenous neurotransmitters to activate neurotransmitter receptors (drug agonist). Other drugs act by antagonizing the binding of endogenous neurotransmitters and inhibiting their effects (drug antagonist). Drugs may also act by altering the synthesis, release, uptake, or degradation of a neurotransmitter. Drug signals are terminated by dissociation of the ligand from the target receptors or enzyme. Chronic psychotropic drug treatment appears to exert its effects through regulation of neuronal signaling elements at a variety of levels, including neurotransmitters, receptors, G proteins, second messengers, protein kinases, transcription factors, and transcription factor–induced gene expression. Chronic drug agonist treatment produces downregulation of receptors by altering receptor recycling or by reducing receptor synthesis. Chronic agonist treatment can produce desensitization of its respective receptor via receptor modification by a protein kinase, resulting in reduction of the receptor's functional effect. These processes oppose the effects of chronic receptor stimulation.

Drugs such as antipsychotics produce effects at a variety of levels, including neurophysiological, neurochemical, molecular, and genomic. At a neurophysiological level, acute antipsychotic treatment activates mesolimbic dopaminergic neurons, whereas chronic antipsychotic drug treatment produces delayed inactivation of dopamine neuronal firing, or depolarization blockade. These chronic drug effects are associated with functional consequences, including akinesia and disruption of reward behaviors in animal models. Chronic treatment with the typical antipsychotic haloperidol produces depolarization blockade of both nigrostriatal and mesocorticolimbic dopaminergic neurons, which are associated with extrapyramidal and therapeutic effects of this agent, respectively (Chiodo and Bunney 1993). Neurophysiological studies show that chronic treatment with an atypical antipsychotic, such as clozapine, reduces the firing of mesocorticolimbic but not nigrostriatal neurons. Blockade of nigrostriatal cells by antipsychotics appears to produce extrapyramidal side effects such as parkinsonism, whereas blockade of mesocorticolimbic cells projecting to the prefrontal cortex and ventral striatum appears to be responsible for the therapeutic effects of these drugs (Grace et al. 1997).

The fact that different brain circuits are activated by typical and atypical antipsychotics probably accounts for their differing clinical and adverse effects. Measuring immediate-early gene responses to antipsychotic drug treatment, such as *c-fos* response, in specific neuroanatomic regions is useful for delineating the circuits that are activated by antipsychotic drugs (Schulman and Hyman 1999). Atypical antipsychotics activate mesocorticolimbic dopaminergic terminal regions, including prefrontal cortical and nucleus accumbens neurons, which are involved in cognition and emotional expression (Robertson et al. 1994). Typical antipsychotic agents activate some mescorticolimbic regions and also the nigrostriatal targets responsible for extrapyramidal side effects (Nguyen et al. 1992). Antipsychotic-induced striatal *c-fos* expression is blocked by CREB antisense oligonucleotide administration in the striatum, suggesting the importance of a cAMP mechanism for antipsychotic actions (Konradi and Heckers 1995).

Different molecular mechanisms operate in typical and atypical antipsychotics, and these likely account for their differing clinical and adverse effects. In part, antipsychotic drugs exert their cellular effects via blockade of D_2-like dopamine receptors. Because D_2 dopamine receptors are negatively coupled to adenylyl cyclase, D_2 receptor antagonists such as haloperidol would be expected to stimulate the synthesis of cAMP. In fact, short-term treatment with typical antipsychotic drugs stimulates adenylyl cyclase activity in cells with D_2-like dopamine receptors (Hall and Strange 1997). Acute haloperidol treatment also produces significant increases in striatal concentrations of downstream effector PKA (Kaplan et al. 2001). Other receptors implicated in antipsychotic drug actions—such as muscarinic cholinergic receptors—are also coupled to adenylyl cyclase. In cells with muscarinic M_4 receptors, atypical antipsychotic drugs such as clozapine inhibit cAMP production, while typical antipsychotics, such as haloperidol, chlorpromazine, and others, have no effect on cAMP in these cells (Zeng et al. 1997). Studies of chronic treatment support the role of cAMP mechanisms:

haloperidol treatment increases adenylyl cyclase activity in medicated subjects versus controls, whereas olanzapine (an atypical antipsychotic) reduces adenylyl cyclase activity in frontal cortex projection areas (Kaplan et al. 1999b). Mice lacking the gene that encodes a regulatory subunit of PKA fail to express haloperidol-induced behavioral responses and activation of nigrostriatal neurons (Adams et al. 1997).

The role of phosphatidylinositol pathways in the mediation of antipsychotic drug actions has also been elucidated. Given that D_2 dopamine receptors are positively coupled to inositol phosphatide hydrolysis, D_2 receptor antagonists would be expected to inhibit this signaling pathway. In fact, acute and chronic administration of typical antipsychotics in rats reduces concentrations of effector enzyme phospholipase C and inhibits production of its second messenger, inositol triphosphate, in the striatum. Similarly, acute and chronic typical antipsychotic treatment reduces the activity and concentrations of the downstream PKC enzyme in the striatum. Atypical antipsychotics have no such effects on D_2-mediated phosphatidylinositol and PKC signaling, again demonstrating differences in molecular mechanisms between the two types of agents (Dwivedi and Pandey 1999).

These effects of typical and atypical antipsychotics on cAMP and phosphoinositol signaling could produce differing downstream effects on PKA and PKC, respectively. Drug-induced regulation of protein kinases alters downstream phosphorylation of the transcription factors CREB (Kaplan et al. 2001) and Fos. Because activation of cAMP pathways induces transcription of the immediate-early gene *c-fos* (Metz and Ziff 1991), typical and atypical antipsychotics could produce their differential effects on *c-fos* expression via cAMP signaling. Antipsychotics regulate protein kinases and their phosphorylation of transcription factors, and this could result in transcriptional alterations in target neurons. Drug-induced changes in the transcription and translation of new proteins in mesocorticolimbic dopaminergic systems may produce long-term adaptations in these neurons that could account for the clinical effects of these agents (see Figure 2–4). In fact, acute treatment with haloperidol has been shown to induce the transcription of an array of mRNAs from multiple genes (Berke et al. 1998).

Conclusions

We have provided only one example of molecular mechanisms of psychiatric drugs in specific neuronal circuits. Much research is needed to determine which molecular changes in mesocorticolimbic neurons are responsible for the cellular and therapeutic effects of antipsychotics.

Such research could ultimately lead to the development of new therapeutic targets and to delineation of the pathophysiology of the underlying disorder. Elucidating signal transduction mechanisms in relevant brain circuitry provides a more refined understanding of psychiatric illness and of current and future treatments.

References

Adams MR, Brandon EP, Chartoff EH, et al: Loss of haloperidol induced gene expression and catalepsy in protein kinase A-deficient mice. Proc Natl Acad Sci U S A 94:12157–12161, 1997

Berke JD, Paletzki RF, Aronson GJ, et al: A complex program of striatal gene expression induced by dopaminergic stimulation. J Neurosci 18:5301–5310, 1998

Bloom FE: Neurotransmission and the central nervous system, in Goodman and Gilman's The Pharmacological Basis of Therapeutic, 9th Edition. Edited by Hardman JG, Limbird LE. New York, McGraw-Hill, 1996, pp 267–294

Boulton AA, Eisenhofer G: Catecholamine metabolism: from molecular understanding to clinical diagnosis and treatment. Adv Pharmacol 42:273–292, 1998

Bowery NG, Enna SJ: Gamma-aminobutyric acid(B) receptors: first of the functional metabotropic heterodimers. J Pharmacol Exp Ther 292:2–7, 2000

Brady S, Colman DR, Brophy P: Subcellular organization of the nervous system: organelles and their functions, in Basic Neurochemistry: Molecular, Cellular and Medical Aspects, 6th Edition. Edited by Siegel GJ, Agranoff BW, Albers RW, et al. Philadelphia, PA, Lippincott-Raven, 1999, pp 71–106

Catterall WA: Structure and function of voltage-gated ion channels. Annu Rev Biochem 65:493–531, 1995

Chiodo LA, Bunney BS: Typical and atypical neuroleptics: differential effects of chronic administration on the activity of A9 and A10 midbrain dopaminergic neurons. J Neurosci 3:1607–1619, 1983

Clapham DE: Calcium signaling. Cell 80:259–268, 1995

De Camilli P, Takei K: Molecular mechanisms in synaptic vesicle endocytosis and recycling. Neuron 16:481–486, 1996

Deutch AY, Roth RH: Neurotransmitters, in Neurobiology of Mental Illness. Edited by Charney DS, Nestler EJ, Bunney BS. New York, Oxford University Press, 1999, pp 193–234

Dingledine R, McBain CJ: Glutamate and aspartate, in Basic Neurochemistry: Molecular, Cellular and Medical Aspects, 6th Edition. Edited by Siegel GJ, Agranoff BW, Albers RW, et al. Philadelphia, PA, Lippincott-Raven, 1999, pp 263–292

Dwivedi Y, Pandey GN: Effects of treatment with haloperidol, chlorpromazine and clozapine on protein kinase C and phosphoinositide-specific phospholipase C activity and on mRNA and protein expression of PKC and PLC isozymes in rat brain. J Pharmacol Exp Ther 291:688–704, 1999

Ferre S: Adenosine-dopamine interactions in the ventral striatum. Implications for the treatment of schizophrenia. Psychopharmacology (Berl) 133:107–120, 1997

Frazer A, Hensler JG: Serotonin, in Basic Neurochemistry: Molecular, Cellular and Medical Aspects, 6th Edition. Edited by Siegel GJ, Agranoff BW, Albers RW, et al. Philadelphia, PA, Lippincott-Raven, 1999, pp 263–292

Girault J-A, Greengard P: Principles of signal transduction, in Neurobiology of Mental Illness. Edited by Charney DS, Nestler EJ, Bunney BS. New York, Oxford University Press, 1999, pp 37–60

Grace AA, Bunney BS, Moore H, et al: Dopamine-cell depolarization block as a model for the therapeutic actions of antipsychotic drugs. Trends Neurosci 20:31–37, 1997

Hall DA, Strange PG: Evidence that antipsychotic drugs are inverse agonists at D2 dopamine receptors. Br J Pharmacol 121:731–736, 1997

Holz RW, Fisher SK: Synaptic transmission and cellular signaling: an overview, in Basic Neurochemistry: Molecular, Cellular and Medical Aspects, 6th Edition. Edited by Siegel GJ, Agranoff BW, Albers RW, et al. Philadelphia, PA, Lippincott-Raven, 1999, pp 213–242

Hyman SE, Nestler EJ: Mechanisms of neural plasticity, in Neurobiology of Mental Illness. Edited by Charney DS, Nestler EJ, Bunney BS. New York, Oxford University Press, 1999, pp 61–72

Jaber M, Robinson SW, Missale C, et al: Dopamine receptors and brain function. Neuropharmacology 35:1503–1519, 1996

Kandel ER, Siegelbaum SA, Schwartz JH: Synaptic transmission, in Principles of Neural Science, 3rd Edition. Edited by Kandel ER, Schwartz JH, Jessell TM. Norwalk, CT, Appleton & Lange, 1990, pp 123–134

Kaplan GB, Sears MT: Adenosine receptor agonists attenuate and adenosine receptor antagonists exacerbate opiate withdrawal signs. Psychopharmacology (Berl) 123:64–70, 1996

Kaplan GB, Bharmal NP, Leite-Morris KA, et al: Role of adenosine A1 and A2a receptors in the alcohol withdrawal syndrome. Alcohol 19:157–162, 1999a

Kaplan GB, Leite-Morris KA, Keith DJ: Differential effects of treatment with typical and atypical antipsychotic drugs on adenylyl cyclase and G proteins. Neurosci Lett 273:147–150, 1999b

Kaplan GB, Turalba AV, Leite-Morris KA: Antipsychotic drug treatment regulates CREB phosphorylation in terminal regions of nigrostriatal and mesocorticolimbic pathways. Society for Neuroscience Abstracts 27:875.12, 2001

Konradi C, Heckers S: Haloperidol-induced Fos expression in striatum is dependent upon transcription factor cyclic AMP response element binding protein. Neuroscience 65:1051–1061, 1995

Kuhar MJ, Coucero PR, Lambert PD: Catecholamines, in Basic Neurochemistry: Molecular, Cellular and Medical Aspects, 6th Edition. Edited by Siegel GJ, Agranoff BW, Albers RW, et al. Philadelphia, PA, Lippincott-Raven, 1999, pp 243–261

Mains RE, Eipper BA: Peptides, in Basic Neurochemistry: Molecular, Cellular and Medical Aspects, 6th Edition. Edited by Siegel GJ, Agranoff BW, Albers RW, et al. Philadelphia, PA, Lippincott-Raven, 1999, pp 363–382

Malenka RC, Nicoll RA: Long-term potentiation—a decade of progress? Science 285:1870–1874, 1999

Manji HK, Potter WZ, Lenox RH: Signal transduction pathways: molecular targets for lithium's actions. Arch Gen Psychiatry 52:531–543, 1995

McCormick DA: Membrane potential and action potential, in Fundamental Neuroscience. Edited by Zigmond MJ, Bloom FE, Landis SC, et al. San Diego, CA, Academic Press, 1999, pp 129–154

Meghji P: Adenosine production and metabolism, in Adenosine in the Nervous System. Edited by Stone TW. San Diego, CA, Academic Press, 1991, pp 25–42

Mehta AK, Ticku MK: An update on GABA-A receptors. Brain Res Brain Res Rev 29:196–217, 1999

Metz R, Ziff E: cAMP stimulates the C/EBP-related transcription factor rNFIL-6 to trans-locate to the nucleus and induce c-fos transcription. Genes Dev 5:1754–1766, 1991

Mochly-Rosen D: Localization of protein kinases by anchoring proteins: a theme in signal transduction. Science 268:247–251, 1995

Murphy DL, Andrews AM, Wichems CH, et al: Brain serotonin neurotransmission: an overview and update with an emphasis on serotonin subsystem heterogeneity, multiple receptors, interactions with other neurotransmitter systems, and consequent implications for understanding the actions of serotonergic drugs. J Clin Psychiatry 59 (suppl 15):4–12, 1998

Neer EJ: Heterotrimeric G proteins: organizers of transmembrane signals. Cell 80:249–257, 1995

Nguyen TV, Kosofsky BE, Birnbaum R, et al: Differential expression of c-fos and zif268 in rat striatum after haloperidol, clozapine, and amphetamine. Proc Natl Acad Sci U S A 89:4270–4274, 1992

Raine CS: Neurocellular anatomy, in Basic Neurochemistry: Molecular, Cellular and Medical Aspects, 6th Edition. Edited by Siegel GJ, Agranoff BW, Albers RW, et al. Philadelphia, PA, Lippincott-Raven, 1999, pp 3–30

Robertson GS, Matsumura H, Fibiger HC: Induction patterns of Fos-like immunoreactivity in the forebrain as predictors of atypical antipsychotic activity. J Pharmacol Exp Ther 271:1058–1066, 1994

Sarter M, Bruno JP: Cognitive functions of cortical acetylcholine: toward a unifying hypothesis. Brain Res Brain Res Rev 23:28–46, 1997

Schulman H, Hyman SE: Intracellular signaling, in Fundamental Neuroscience. Edited by Zigmond MJ, Bloom FE, Landis SC, et al. San Diego, CA, Academic Press, 1999, pp 269–316

Waxman MN: Neurotransmitter receptors, in Fundamental Neuroscience. Edited by Zigmond MJ, Bloom FE, Landis SC, et al. San Diego, CA, Academic Press, 1999, pp 235–268

Zeng XP, Le F, Richelson E: Muscarinic m4 receptor activation by some atypical antipsychotic drugs. Eur J Pharmacol 321:349–354, 1997

CHAPTER 3

Neural Circuitry and Signaling in Schizophrenia

Stephan Heckers, M.D.
Donald C. Goff, M.D.

Clinical Presentation

The psychiatric diagnoses *dementia praecox* (defined by Emil Kraepelin) and *group of schizophrenias* (defined by Eugen Bleuler) were introduced to designate a group of psychiatric patients with similar clinical features, disease course, and outcome (Hoenig 1995). The diagnostic criteria used to define schizophrenia have varied over the last 100 years. They have included several forms of hallucinations and delusions, abnormalities of speech and behavior, cognitive deficits such as poor attention and impaired memory, and affective disturbance (Alpert 1985). Schizophrenia is now diagnosed in about 1% of the population worldwide.

In the fifth edition of his psychiatry textbook, published in 1896, Kraepelin proposed that three groups of patients, diagnosed with catatonia, hebephrenia, and dementia paranoides, represent different phenotypes of a single illness that he labeled *dementia praecox* (Palha and Esteves 1997). Furthermore, he proposed that dementia praecox is separate from manic-depressive illness, in part because of a poorer prognosis. During the first decade of the twentieth century, Kraepelin revised his dichotomy of psychotic illness and added paranoia and paraphrenia as separate diagnoses. We are still struggling to answer the two questions Kraepelin faced 100 years ago: How is schizophrenia different from other psychotic conditions? Is schizophrenia one illness, or does it represent different diseases?

There is general agreement that psychotic states associated with drug use or medical illness (i.e., secondary psychoses) are fundamentally different from psychotic states without clear precipitating factors (i.e., psychotic disorders). The secondary psychoses might inform us about the neural mechanisms of psychotic symptoms, but they do not necessarily provide clues to the pathology of psychotic disorders. There is much less agreement about the classification of the psychotic illnesses. The theoretical spectrum ranges from the view that there are no disease entities, only continua of variation (Crow 1986); to Kraepelin's classical dichotomy; to the current DSM-IV-TR (American Psychiatric Association 2000) classification of six separate psychotic disorders (delusional disorder, schizophreniform disorder, schizophrenia, schizoaffective disorder, psychotic depression, and bipolar disorder); and finally to elaborate classifications of more than 20 different types of psychosis (Leonhard 1995).

How is schizophrenia diagnosed? First, the diagnosis can be made if specific inclusion criteria are met. Kurt Schneider proposed first-rank criteria, relating to the nature of auditory hallucinations, to discriminate schizophrenia from other psychotic illnesses (Schneider 1959), and these criteria were included in several classification schemes. Second, certain qualifiers make schizophrenia distinct from other psychotic illnesses: greater than 6 months' duration of symptoms, no prominent mood symptoms, and no medical illness or drug use precipitating the psychotic symptoms. These qualifiers are designed to increase the reliability of the schizophrenia diagnosis. Reliability of a clinical diagnosis is defined as the likelihood that a given patient will consistently receive the same diagnosis when rated by the same (intrarater) or a different (interrater) clinician. Inconsistent definitions of schizophrenia previously had resulted in markedly different rates of schizophrenia diagnoses (Kendell et al. 1971), but with the use of qualifiers and the inclusion of two first-rank symptoms, the diagnosis of schizophrenia has now become one of the most reliable diagnoses in all of psychiatry (Sartorius et al. 1995). The qualifiers function as gatekeepers: they separate schizophrenia from conditions that might present with the same symptoms but are less severe, are briefer, or are due to another illness.

Good reliability of the diagnosis does not ensure that schizophrenia represents an actual disease entity. Diagnostic entities should predict course, treatment response, and outcome. The schizophrenia diagnosis predicts none of these. First, the polythetic definition of schizophrenia creates a heterogeneous clinical picture: any two of a total of five different symptoms suffice to fulfill criteria for the DSM-IV-TR diagnosis of schizophrenia. Various permutations of these symptoms can give rise to the diagnosis of schizophrenia. Second, the course and outcome of the disease are highly variable and seem to fall into three categories: episodic—good outcome; chronic—moderate impairment; and chronic—poor outcome. Third, the response to treatment is associated with several factors—such as gender, premorbid function, and comorbidity—but does not follow a predictable pattern.

Subtyping Schizophrenia

The heterogeneity of the schizophrenia construct poses a major hurdle for the study of disease mechanisms and etiology. If the diagnosis covers a broad spectrum of patients who might not share the same symptoms, the search for one etiology and pathogenesis that could predict treatment response and outcome may be futile. Therefore, schizophrenia researchers have attempted to reduce the complexity of schizophrenia by defining subtypes or dividing schizophrenia into one or more entities.

Emil Kraepelin divided dementia praecox into subtypes based on the presence of one or more symptoms. His last attempt at subdividing dementia praecox/schizophrenia produced 10 different "clinical forms" (Kraepelin 1919). The American Psychiatric Association's *Diagnostic and Statistical Manual of Mental Disorders* has followed his tradition; the current edition (DSM-IV-TR) recognizes three of Kraepelin's subtypes (paranoid type, disorganized or hebephrenic type, catatonic type) and supplements these with two new ones (undifferentiated type, residual type). Although these Kraepelinian subtypes are defined by the presence, severity, and duration of symptoms, their validity has been questioned. For example, poor temporal stability is seen in all of Kraepelin's subtypes except paranoid type and thus might not represent a trait characteristic (Fenton and McGlashan 1991).

A different approach to the complexity of schizophrenia can be traced back to the writings of John Russell Reynolds (1828–1896) and John Hughlings Jackson (1835–1911). Jackson proposed a model of abnormal brain function in neurological and psychiatric disorders based on the theory that the brain had evolved to increasingly more complex levels. He suggested that higher levels of brain function (e.g., cortex) control the function of lower levels (e.g., subcortical structures, brain stem). Negative symptoms arise from the paralysis of a given hypothetical level of brain function. Positive symptoms arise when higher levels of brain function are impaired and, due to a lack of inhibition, lower levels become apparent, creating "symptoms" normally not observed (Berrios 1985).

The positive/negative dichotomy resonated in the community of schizophrenia researchers. It seemed reasonable to divide the signs and symptoms of schizophrenia into those characterized by the production of abnormal behavior (positive symptoms) and those representing a deficiency of normal behavior (negative symptoms). It was thought that the two symptom dimensions could differentiate subtypes of schizophrenia. Positive symptoms include hallucinations, delusions, thought disorder, and bizarre behaviors. Negative symptoms include alogia, affective blunting, avolition, anhedonia, and attentional impairment (Greden and Tandon 1991).

Localizing Schizophrenia Symptoms

Once subtypes of schizophrenia had been defined, researchers attempted to localize the clinical features to distinct brain regions or neural networks. Southard published one of the first such models, proposing that temporal lesions (especially left superior temporal gyrus hypoplasia) are associated with auditory hallucinations, parietal atrophy and sclerosis are associated with catatonia, and frontal lobe aplasia or atrophy is associated with delusions (Southard 1914).

More recently, the positive and negative symptoms have been linked to dysfunction of separate neural networks (Liddle et al. 1992). For example, positive symptoms of schizophrenia have been correlated with temporal lobe abnormalities such as volume reduction and increased blood flow. Conversely, negative symptoms have been associated with decreased prefrontal blood flow.

Carpenter and colleagues suggested that schizophrenia patients can be classified either as deficit-syndrome patients, who have enduring negative symptoms that are not due to medication and/or depression, or as nondeficit patients. They proposed that deficit patients show more frontal lobe deficits than do nondeficit patients but that both subgroups show temporal lobe abnormalities (Carpenter et al. 1993). So far, studies have reported differential impairment of cognitive function (Buchanan et al. 1997), brain structure (Buchanan et al. 1993), and brain function (Tamminga et al. 1992) in deficit and nondeficit schizophrenia.

Localizing the signs and symptoms of schizophrenia to neural networks relies on neuroscientific models of how behavior is implemented in the brain. In the next section we present a basic outline of brain-behavior relationships. We then use this framework to review studies of the neural basis of schizophrenia.

Neural Circuitry

The underlying premise in the definition of psychosis is that the brain's processing of information derived from the outside world is perturbed. The processing of sensory information involves three steps: the collection of sensory information through perceptual modules, the creation of a representation, and the production of a response.

Sensory organs provide information about physical attributes of objects and events. Details of physical attributes (e.g., temperature, sound frequency, color) are conveyed through multiple segregated channels within each perceptual module. Integration of the highly segregated sensory information occurs at three levels. The first integration occurs in unimodal association areas where physical attributes of one sensory domain are linked together. A second level of integration is reached in multimodal association areas, which link physical attributes of different sensory qualities together. A third level of integration is provided by the interpretation and evaluation of experience. At this third level of integration, the brain creates a representation of experience that has the spatiotemporal resolution and full complexity of the outside world. Building on previous theoretical efforts (Goldman-Rakic 1987), we propose that the positive (psychotic) symptoms are due to an imbalance in the generation of representations. We further suggest that these symptoms are generated by 1) impairment of the ability to classify representations as internally or externally generated (in the case of hallucinations) and 2) immutable linking of representations with each other in the absence of external dependency (in the case of delusions).

Following the evaluation and interpretation of the representation, the brain creates a response through a variety of channels (e.g., language, affect, motor behavior). The diagnosis of psychosis is based on the analysis of these responses. For example, hallucinations, delusions, formal thought disorder, and flat affect are defined by abnormalities of the patient's language and motor behavior.

Several anatomic systems are involved in higher-order information processing. We limit our discussion here to four anatomic systems: the cortex, the thalamus, the basal ganglia, and the medial temporal lobe (Figure 3–1). First, we provide an overview of how these anatomic systems work together during normal brain function. We then review, in detail, each of the four systems and how they are perturbed in psychosis.

The thalamus is the gateway to cortical processing for all incoming sensory information, here represented by the three major systems: somatosensory, auditory, and visual. Primary sensory cortical areas (S1, A1, V1) receive sensory information from the appropriate sensory modules (sensory organ + thalamus). To create the representation of experience, the association cortex integrates information from primary cortices, from subcortical structures, and from brain areas affiliated with memory. The medial temporal lobe serves two major functions in the brain: to integrate multimodal sensory information for storage into and retrieval from memory, and to attach limbic valence to sensory information. The basal ganglia are primarily involved in the integration of input from cortical areas, particularly from the motor cortex. They modulate the activity of thalamocortical projections, thereby creating a cortico-striato-pallido-thalamo-cortical loop.

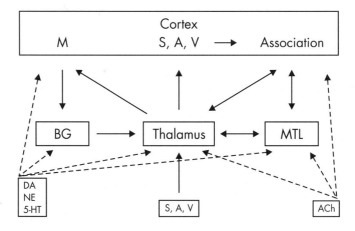

Circuitry	Psychosis models			
	Glu	DA	MTL	DLPFC
1) S, A, V → Thalamus → Cortex (S, A, V)	+			
2) Cortex → BG → Thalamus → Cortex	+	+		
3) Cortex → MTL	+	+	+	+
4) Cortex → MTL → Thalamus → Cortex	+	+	+	+

Figure 3–1. *Basic circuitry of information processing in the human brain.* **Solid arrows** *indicate glutamatergic pathways.* **Broken arrows** *indicate the widespread, neurotransmitter-specific projections arising from the basal forebrain (ACh) and brain stem (DA, NE, 5-HT). The basal ganglia–thalamus projection is GABAergic. A = auditory cortex; M = motor cortex; S = sensory cortex; V = visual cortex; GABA = γ-aminobutyric acid; BG = basal ganglia; MTL = medial temporal lobe; DA = dopamine; NE = norepinephrine; 5-HT = 5-hydroxytryptamine (serotonin); ACh = acetylcholine; Glu = glutamate; DLPFC = dorsolateral prefrontal cortex.*

Four groups of densely packed neurons provide widespread projections to many brain areas: cholinergic neurons in the basal forebrain and brain stem, dopaminergic neurons in the substantia nigra and ventral tegmental area, noradrenergic neurons in the locus coeruleus, and serotonergic neurons in the raphe nuclei.

The anatomic organization of the human brain, as outlined in Figure 3–1, gives rise to several neural circuits, each affiliated with different aspects of brain function. Over the last 100 years of psychosis research, four major hypotheses have been put forward that propose abnormalities of these neural circuits in psychosis:

1. Beginning with Kraepelin, psychosis was thought to be a dysfunction of the association cortex in the frontal lobe, the dorsolateral prefrontal cortex (DLPFC).
2. Based in part on the observation that temporal lobe seizures often present with hallucinations and delusions, abnormalities of the medial temporal lobe were proposed to explain the positive symptoms of psychosis.
3. The occurrence of psychotic symptoms after the use of amphetamine and cocaine and the discovery that antipsychotic drugs block dopamine D_2 receptors gave rise to the dopamine hypothesis.
4. More recently, the glutamatergic hypothesis, based in part on the fact that N-methyl-D-aspartate (NMDA) receptor antagonists such as ketamine and phencyclidine can cause drug-induced psychotic states, has been put forward.

We review here the evidence that the four anatomic systems (the cortex, the thalamus, the basal ganglia, and the medial temporal lobe) and their modulation by the neurotransmitter-specific projection systems are abnormal in schizophrenia. Although other brain regions have also been implicated in the pathology of schizophrenia, space does not permit their discussion here.

Cortex

The association cortex of the human brain is a six-layered isocortex (Figure 3–2). Layers 2 and 4 are defined by a high density of small interneurons (i.e., neurons that do not send long-ranging projections to other cortical or subcortical areas). In contrast, layers 3 and 5 are defined by a high density of pyramidal cells, which collect input through their dendrites and project to other cortical or subcortical areas. Interneurons are γ-aminobutyric acid (GABA)ergic cells and exert an inhibitory influence on their targets (via $GABA_A$ receptors), whereas pyramidal cells are glutamatergic and have an excitatory influence. Normal cortical function depends on an intricate balance of GABAergic inhibition and glutamatergic excitation.

Neuronal Architecture

The anatomic and functional organization of the association cortex, especially the DLPFC, has been studied extensively in schizophrenia. Volume reduction of the association cortex in schizophrenia has been reported in several postmortem and neuroimaging studies. However, there is no marked loss of neurons or increased gliosis, a marker for the degeneration of neurons (Heckers 1997).

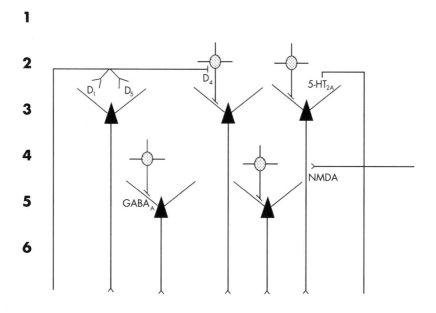

Figure 3–2.   *Schematic diagram of cortical pyramidal neurons (solid), nonpyramidal neurons **(shaded)**, their receptors, and the afferent fiber network. The pyramidal neurons of the cerebral cortex project to other areas, including cortical, subcortical (e.g., thalamus and striatum), and brain stem/spinal cord regions. They receive projections from other cortical areas and from the thalamus. The nonpyramidal neurons of each cortical area modulate their neighboring pyramidal cells via inhibitory GABA$_A$ receptors. Pyramidal and nonpyramidal cortical neurons receive input from widespread projecting neurotransmitter systems of the basal forebrain and brain stem (e.g., dopaminergic and serotonergic neurons). The numbers on the **left side** designate the six layers of isocortex. The effects of these neurotransmitters are conveyed via a variety of postsynaptic receptors on nonpyramidal (e.g., D$_4$) and pyramidal neurons (e.g., D$_1$, D$_5$). D$_1$, D$_4$, D$_5$ = dopamine receptors; 5-HT = 5-hydroxytryptamine (serotonin); GABA = γ-aminobutyric acid; NMDA = N-methyl-D-aspartate.*

Several subtle yet significant changes of the cortical architecture have been reported. First, a small subset of cortical neurons that express the enzyme nicotinamide adenine dinucleotide phosphate-diaphorase (NADPH-d) has been found to be reduced in the frontal and temporal cortex and increased in number in the underlying white matter (Akbarian et al. 1993). Similarly, the distribution of the Cajal-Retzius cells is shifted to lower parts of the first cortical layer (Kalus et al. 1997). Second, increased cell density in the frontal and occipital cortices has been described and attributed to changes in cortical neuropil (Selemon et al.

1995). Third, several abnormalities of GABAergic interneurons have been described: reduced release and uptake of GABA at synaptic terminals (Simpson et al. 1989), decreased expression of the GABA-synthesizing enzyme glutamic acid decarboxylase (GAD) (Akbarian et al. 1995), altered expression of $GABA_A$ receptors (Benes et al. 1996b), and a reduction of axon cartridges of GABAergic chandelier neurons that terminate on the initial segment of pyramidal cell axons (Woo et al. 1998). Fourth, the dendritic organization of frontal cortical areas has been found to be abnormal (Garey et al. 1998). Finally, the organization of synaptic connections, studied with the growth-associated protein GAP-43, has been found to be abnormal in frontal and visual association cortices (Perrone-Bizzozero et al. 1996).

Neurotransmitter Systems

Cortical neurons are targets for ascending fibers arising from the underlying white matter. Some of these inputs originate from other cortical areas or from the thalamus. Others—such as the dopaminergic neurons of the ventral tegmental area and the serotonergic neurons of the raphe nuclei—arise from neurotransmitter-specific projection systems. Modulation of cortical function via the dopamine D_1, D_4, and D_5 receptors and 5-hydroxytryptamine (5-HT) 2A receptors leads to the "fine tuning" of information processing—for example, by increasing the signal-to-noise ratio during corticocortical and thalamocortical neurotransmission (Goldman-Rakic 1998).

The effect of dopamine on cortical neurons is transduced by three dopamine receptors, namely the D_1, D_4, and D_5 receptors. The D_1 and D_5 receptors are expressed primarily, but not exclusively (Muly et al. 1998), on pyramidal cells, whereas the D_4 receptor is expressed primarily on GABAergic interneurons (Mrzljak et al. 1996). Compared with typical antipsychotics, which have a high D_2-blocking ability, the atypical antipsychotics are much more effective in blocking D_4 receptors. It is not clear whether some of the antipsychotic effects of atypical antipsychotics are conveyed through the D_4 receptors localized on GABAergic interneurons of the association cortex, especially the DLPFC (Lidow et al. 1998).

Alterations of the GABAergic system (Akbarian et al. 1995; Benes et al. 1996b) and of the D_1 receptors of the DLPFC have been reported in schizophrenia. The expression of cortical D_1 receptors is increased by chronic treatment with typical antipsychotics (Knable et al. 1996). Of interest, a recent positron-emission tomography (PET) study found a reduction of cortical D_1 receptors that correlated with the severity of negative symptoms and poor performance on the Wisconsin Card Sorting Test (Okubo et al. 1997).

One serotonergic receptor, the 5-HT$_{2A}$ subtype, is of relevance for the pathophysiology of psychosis (Jakab and Goldman-Rakic 1998). Hallucinogens (e.g., lysergic acid diethylamide [LSD]) act as agonists at the 5-HT$_{2A}$ receptor, and several antipsychotic compounds, especially the atypical antipsychotics, block the activity of the 5-HT$_{2A}$ receptor. Although some postmortem studies have reported a decrease of 5-HT$_{2A}$ receptors in schizophrenia, others have not (for a review, see Lewis et al. 1999). A recent PET study of antipsychotic-free schizophrenia patients did not find any differences in the expression of cortical 5-HT$_{2A}$ receptors in several cortical areas (Lewis et al. 1999).

Cortical Function

Neuroimaging studies have revealed dysfunctional cortical networks in schizophrenia (Gur 1995). Regional cerebral blood flow (rCBF) and glucose metabolism were found to be abnormal in frontal cortical and temporal lobe structures at rest as well as during the performance of cognitive tasks. There is, however, no pattern that is diagnostic for schizophrenia. For example, frontal cortical neuronal activity was found to be lower in schizophrenia patients than in healthy control subjects in some studies (Weinberger et al. 1986) but not in others (Gur et al. 1983; Mathew et al. 1982). Temporal lobe activity at rest was reduced (Gur et al. 1987), normal (Volkow et al. 1987), or increased (Gur et al. 1995) in schizophrenic subjects in different studies. Similarly, frontal cortical recruitment during task performance was reduced in some studies (Weinberger et al. 1986).

The clinical heterogeneity of schizophrenia might explain why schizophrenia as a whole is not associated with a pathognomonic abnormality of brain function. When the signs and symptoms of schizophrenia are used to categorize patients into two groups (positive and negative syndrome) or into distinct clusters, a more consistent pattern of neural dysfunction in schizophrenia emerges. Frontal cortical activity at rest correlates inversely with the degree of negative symptoms (Liddle et al. 1992; Volkow et al. 1987), and left medial temporal lobe activity at rest correlates positively with the severity of psychopathology (DeLisi et al. 1989) and the degree of reality distortion (Liddle et al. 1992). Similarly, decreased frontal cortex recruitment during the performance of some cognitive tasks occurs primarily in patients with negative symptoms (Andreasen et al. 1992).

Thalamus

The thalamus serves several important functions in information processing in the human brain. First, the relay nuclei (the ventral posterior lateral nucleus, medial geniculate nucleus, and lateral geniculate nucleus) relay sensory information from the sensory organs to the appropriate areas of the primary sensory cortex (S1, A1, and V1, respectively) (Figure 3–3). Second, the association nuclei, especially the mediodorsal nucleus, establish reciprocal connections with the association cortex. Third, the motor nuclei (ventral) relay input from the basal ganglia to the motor and premotor cortex (Scheibel 1997).

Two abnormalities of thalamic function have been proposed in schizophrenia. First, breakdown of the sensory filter may lead to an increased stimulation of primary sensory cortical areas. Such a defective filter would implicate abnormalities in the thalamic relay nuclei. Second, dysfunction of the mediodorsal nucleus may lead to impairments of cortical association areas, especially the DLPFC.

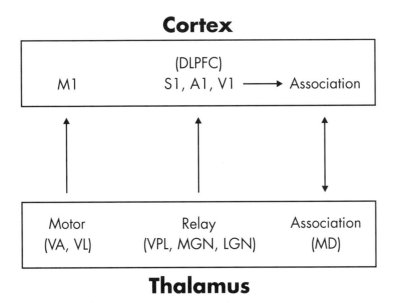

Cortex

(DLPFC)		
M1	S1, A1, V1 ——▶	Association

Motor	Relay	Association
(VA, VL)	(VPL, MGN, LGN)	(MD)

Thalamus

Figure 3–3.   *Three functional subdivisions of the human thalamus. Somatosensory information is relayed via the ventral posterior lateral nucleus (VPL), auditory information via the medial geniculate nucleus (MGN), and visual information via the lateral geniculate nucleus (LGN) to the appropriate primary cortices. Association areas of the cerebral cortex establish reciprocal connections with the mediodorsal (MD) nucleus, and motor information travels from the striatum via the ventral anterior (VA) and ventral lateral (VL) nuclei to the motor cortex (M1). A1 = primary auditory cortex; DLPFC = dorsolateral prefrontal cortex; M1 = primary motor cortex; S1 = primary sensory cortex; V1 = primary visual cortex.*

Direct evidence for an involvement of the thalamus in the patho-physiology of schizophrenia is still limited. The most convincing evidence comes from morphometric studies pointing to a volume reduction of the thalamus, especially the mediodorsal nucleus, which has been attributed to cell loss (Heckers 1997; Pakkenberg 1990). A postmortem study reported a decrease of parvalbumin-positive neurons in the anteroventral nucleus that could result in loss of thalamocortical projections to the prefrontal cortex (Danos et al. 1998). Some (Andreasen et al. 1994) but not all (Portas et al. 1998) neuroimaging studies have revealed smaller thalamic volumes in schizophrenic subjects. In addition, thalamic metabolism and blood flow were found to be impaired at rest and during the performance of cognitive tasks (Hazlett et al. 1999). Of interest in that study, the decrease of metabolism during the performance of a serial verbal learning test involved primarily the region of the mediodorsal thalamic nucleus.

Basal Ganglia

The basal ganglia include the ventral striatum, the dorsal striatum (caudate and putamen), and the globus pallidus (Figure 3–4). The dorsal striatum (caudate, putamen) receives input from several areas of the cerebral cortex and projects to the globus pallidus. The globus pallidus relays the neostriatal input to the thalamus. The thalamus, in turn, projects back to the cortical areas that gave rise to the cortico-striatal projections, thereby closing the cortico-striato-pallido-thalamo-cortical loop. This loop is involved in the generation and control of motor behavior (via connections to the motor cortex) and several cognitive functions (via connections to the association cortex). In contrast, the ventral striatum (the nucleus accumbens) is connected with the amygdala, hippocampus, and hypothalamus and is therefore considered part of the limbic system. Reward and expectancy behavior and their derailment during drug addiction involve the recruitment of the nucleus accumbens.

All basal ganglia structures are modulated by neurotransmitter-specific projection systems, in particular by dopaminergic neurons. Dopaminergic neurons of the substantia nigra project to the neostriatum (nigrostriatal fibers), and dopaminergic neurons of the ventral tegmental area project to the nucleus accumbens (mesolimbic fibers) and cortex (mesocortical fibers). The two major dopamine receptors in the dorsal striatum are the D_1 and D_2 receptors. The nucleus accumbens expresses these receptors and the D_3 receptor.

The basal ganglia are important in psychosis research in three ways: 1) as potential sites of antipsychotic drug action at D_2 receptors, 2) as a

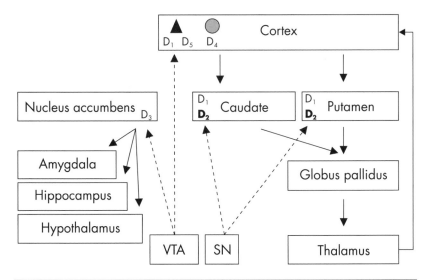

Figure 3–4. *Connectivity and dopaminergic innervation of the neostriatum and limbic striatum. The dopaminergic neurons of the substantia nigra (SN) project to neurons of the neostriatum, which mainly express D_1 and D_2 receptors. The dopaminergic neurons of the ventral tegmental area (VTA) project to neurons in the nucleus accumbens; neurons in this projection area express a high density of D_3 receptors. The dopaminergic neurons of the VTA also project to the cortex, where pyramidal neurons and nonpyramidal neurons express primarily three dopamine receptor types, the D_1, D_5, and D_4 receptors.*

site for the generation of abnormal motor behavior during psychosis (e.g., catatonia), and 3) as a site for pathology in the limbic system (Lidsky 1997).

Dopaminergic Afferents

The most extensive research has been at the level of dopamine receptors. Earlier studies reported an increased expression of D_2 receptors, but there is now good agreement from most studies that the D_2 receptor density is not abnormal in schizophrenia (Sedvall and Farde 1995). One fairly recent study reported an increased expression of dopamine D_3 receptors in the nucleus accumbens (Gurevich et al. 1997).

In addition to studies of dopamine receptors, recent studies have examined dopamine release and intrasynaptic dopamine levels in the striatum. Two groups of investigators have independently reported that intrasynaptic levels of dopamine after treatment with amphetamine is increased in schizophrenia (Breier et al. 1997; Laruelle et al. 1996). Thus, not a tonic increase of dopamine release but rather an increased phasic release of dopamine might be involved in the pathophysiology of schizophrenia. In addition, the regulation of striatal dopamine activity via afferent fibers originating in the prefrontal cortex is impaired (Bertolino et al. 1999).

Striatal Structure

Several structural abnormalities of the basal ganglia in schizophrenia have been reported. First, the volume of basal ganglia structures is increased in medicated schizophrenic patients (Heckers et al. 1991b). Striatal volume increase is closely related to treatment with typical antipsychotics: basal ganglia volume is normal or even decreased in newly diagnosed antipsychotic-naïve patients (Keshavan et al. 1998), increases over time during treatment with typical agents, and decreases after patients have been switched to atypical agents (Chakos et al. 1994). The mechanism of this relationship is not clear. Second, recent postmortem studies have provided evidence for an overall increased number of striatal neurons in schizophrenia (Beckmann and Lauer 1997) and for a change in the synaptic organization of the striatum, particularly the caudate nucleus (Kung et al. 1998). Third, the number of nucleus accumbens neurons has been found to be reduced (Pakkenberg 1990).

Medial Temporal Lobe

The medial temporal lobe contains the amygdala, the hippocampal region, and superficial cortical areas that cover the hippocampal region and form the parahippocampal gyrus. The hippocampal region can be subdivided into three subregions: the dentate gyrus, the cornu Ammonis sectors, and the subiculum (Figure 3–5). The neurons of the human hippocampal region are arranged in one cellular layer, the pyramidal cell layer. Most pyramidal cell layer neurons are glutamatergic, whereas the small contingent of nonpyramidal cells is GABAergic. The serial circuitry of glutamatergic neurons provides the structural basis for long-term potentiation, a physiological phenomenon crucial for formation of memory.

The parahippocampal gyrus receives many projections from multimodal cortical association areas and relays them to the hippocampal region (Van Hoesen 1982). Intrinsic connections within the hippocampal region allow further processing before the information is referred back to the association cortex. The hippocampus is also closely connected with the limbic system. On the basis of these connections, Papez (1937)

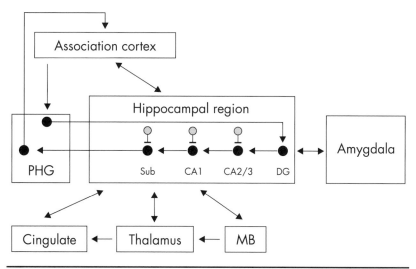

Figure 3–5. *Major connections of the hippocampal region. Neurons from the association cortex project to the dentate gyrus (DG) of the hippocampus via the parahippocampal gyrus (PHG). A serial circuit of glutamatergic neurons in the DG, the cornu Ammonis subfields CA2/3 and CA1, and the subiculum (Sub) processes the cortical information received from the PHG. This information returns to the PHG and the association cortex. The processing of sensory information within the hippocampal region can be modulated via reciprocal connections with components of the limbic system (amygdala, cingulate cortex, thalamus, and mammillary bodies [MB]).*

proposed that the hippocampal formation plays a role in regulating emotion and modulating information processing by attaching limbic valence to sensory stimuli.

In contrast to the century-long search for cortical pathology in schizophrenia, studies of the medial temporal lobe in schizophrenia are just beginning. Nonetheless, an extensive body of research has rapidly accumulated. In the following section we review the evidence for abnormalities of the hippocampal formation in schizophrenia.

Hippocampal Structure

Many studies have found a subtle (about 5%) hippocampal and parahippocampal volume reduction in schizophrenia (McCarley et al. 1999). Hippocampal volume reduction does not correlate with the duration of illness (Velakoulis et al. 1999) or correspond with schizophrenia subtypes such as deficit and nondeficit forms (Buchanan et al. 1993). In addition to changes in volume, changes in hippocampal shape have recently been reported (Csernansky et al. 1998). Furthermore, abnormalities in hippocampal structure are also found in healthy first-degree relatives of schizophrenic patients (Callicott et al. 1998).

Most studies have found no change in the number of hippocampal pyramidal neurons in schizophrenia (Heckers et al. 1991a), but nonpyramidal cells in the hippocampus (especially in the CA2 subregion) seem to be reduced by 40% (Benes et al. 1998). Findings from studies of the orientation and position of pyramidal cells within the cornu Ammonis subfields and of entorhinal cortex layer 2 cells are inconclusive (Arnold et al. 1991). There is evidence that the intrinsic hippocampal fiber systems and the reciprocal connections of the hippocampal formation are perturbed in schizophrenia, leading to a loss of neuropil and an overall loss of white matter (Heckers et al. 1991a). Synaptic organization is changed in the hippocampus in schizophrenic patients, indicating altered neural plasticity in this disorder (Eastwood et al. 1995). In addition to these postmortem studies, magnetic resonance spectroscopy studies have provided evidence for abnormalities of membrane phospholipids and high-energy phosphate metabolism in the temporal lobe (Kegeles et al. 1998).

Neurotransmitter Systems

Glutamate receptors of the kainate/α-amino-3-hydroxy-5-methyl-4-isoxalone propionic acid (KA/AMPA) subtype, primarily the $GluR_1$ and $GluR_2$ subunits, are decreased in the hippocampus in schizophrenia (Eastwood and Harrison 1995; Eastwood et al. 1995). GABA uptake sites are reduced and $GABA_A$ receptors are upregulated, possibly as a result of the loss of GABAergic hippocampal interneurons (Benes et al. 1996a; Selemon et al. 1995). In addition, serotonergic $5\text{-}HT_{1A}$ and $5\text{-}HT_2$ receptors are increased and 5-HT uptake sites are unchanged in the hippocampus in schizophrenia (Joyce et al. 1993).

Hippocampal Function

The metabolism and blood flow of the hippocampus are increased at rest in schizophrenia (Kawasaki et al. 1992). Furthermore, hippocampal and parahippocampal rCBF is increased during psychotic episodes and correlates with positive symptoms (delusions, hallucinations) (Silbersweig et al. 1995). We recently showed that hippocampal recruitment during the conscious recollection of semantically encoded words is impaired in schizophrenia (Heckers et al. 1998). Schizophrenic patients displayed increased levels of hippocampal blood flow at rest and lacked the normal modulation that predicted recall accuracy in control subjects. In addition, indirect evidence (Weinberger et al. 1992) exists for the contribution of hippocampal abnormalities to the cognitive impairments seen in schizophrenia.

Hippocampal Lesion Models of Schizophrenia

Additional evidence for the contribution of hippocampal dysfunction to the pathogenesis of schizophrenia is provided by hippocampal lesion studies in rodents and primates. Hippocampal lesions produce behavioral states that resemble some of those observed in schizophrenia—for example, attentional and memory deficits, stereotypical behavior, hyperarousal, and behavioral changes—but are reversible with antipsychotic drug treatment (Schmajuk 1987). The utility of lesion models has been established in rats (Port et al. 1991) and in nonhuman primates (Saunders et al. 1998)

Signaling Pathways

The Dopamine Model

It has long been recognized that two classes of drugs, the psychostimulants (amphetamines, methylphenidate, and cocaine) and the NMDA receptor antagonists (phencyclidine and ketamine), can produce syndromes resembling schizophrenia in healthy individuals (Goff and Wine 1997). Stimulant psychosis, which has been best studied with amphetamines, is characterized by paranoid delusions; ideas of reference; visual, auditory, or olfactory hallucinations; and agitation—all occurring in the presence of a clear sensorium (Ellinwood 1967). Long-term abuse of amphetamines is associated with apathy and withdrawal (Machiyama 1992). Early studies indicated that many healthy subjects develop psychotic symptoms if administered high doses of amphetamine over several days (Bell 1973). In contrast, approximately half of patients with schizophrenia will exhibit psychotic exacerbation following administration of relatively low doses of stimulant that typically do not produce psychosis in healthy individuals (Janowsky et al. 1973). Additionally, psychotic exacerbation with methylphenidate predicts a more rapid relapse following antipsychotic discontinuation in schizophrenic patients (Lieberman et al. 1984).

Sensitization to behavioral effects is an important characteristic of stimulant abuse. In animal studies, sensitization is defined as increased behavioral response with repeated exposure to a stimulus (usually the stimulus is an environmental stressor or a pharmacological challenge).

In the case of stimulant psychosis, abusing individuals over time develop psychotic symptoms in response to stimulant doses lower than those used in the initial phase of abuse. Sato (1986) observed that sensitization to methamphetamine-induced psychosis can be long lasting: even after many years of abstinence, a single dose of methamphetamine or an environmental stressor may trigger psychosis in an abstinent abuser with a history of sensitization to methamphetamine. As recently reviewed by Lieberman and colleagues (1997), a sensitization model applied to schizophrenia can account for the course of illness, progression of symptoms, and reactivity to environmental factors.

As described earlier, altered dopamine receptor density or abnormal brain concentrations of dopamine and its metabolites in schizophrenia have not been consistently established (Lieberman and Koreen 1993). More compelling have been links between dopamine and negative symptoms (Goff and Evins 1998). Low concentrations of dopamine in cerebrospinal fluid (CSF) (Bowers 1974) and decreased density of D_1 receptors in the prefrontal cortex (Okubo et al. 1997) have been found to correlate with severity of negative symptoms and impairment in performance on tests of prefrontal cortical function. Similarly, dopamine agonists have been shown to improve negative symptoms and performance on tasks that require prefrontal cortical function (Angrist et al. 1982). Improvement of negative symptoms with amphetamine was not blocked by D_2 antagonist treatment (Van Kammen and Boronow 1988). In contrast, stimulants precipitate psychosis in healthy subjects, and this effect can be blocked by D_2 antagonist treatment (Angrist and Lee 1974).

Pycock and colleagues (1980) demonstrated an inverse relationship between mesocortical and mesolimbic dopamine activity in a study in which increased activation of subcortical dopamine was found in rats with lesioned prefrontal cortical dopamine terminals. These findings have led to a dopamine model of schizophrenia that postulates that hypoactivity of mesocortical dopamine transmission in the prefrontal cortex, mediated by D_1 receptors, underlies negative symptoms, whereas hyperactivity of dopamine in mesolimbic pathways, mediated by D_2 receptors, underlies psychotic symptoms (Davis et al. 1991). A further refinement of this model distinguishes between phasic dopamine release, which is mediated by ventral tegmental dopamine neurons in response to environmental stimuli, and tonic release, which is mediated by presynaptic autoreceptors and establishes baseline dopaminergic sensitivity (Grace 1991). Diminished tonic release of dopamine in the cortex is hypothesized to result in supersensitivity of postsynaptic dopaminergic receptors and excessive activation in response to phasic release of dopamine. As previously described, several investigators have found evidence for increased dopamine release in the striatum of schizophrenia patients following acute administration of a stimulant (Breier et al. 1997; Laruelle et al. 1996).

The Glutamate Model

Studies of NMDA receptor antagonists have led to a second pharmacological model for schizophrenia, the glutamate model (Goff and Wine 1997; Javitt and Zukin 1991). It has been recognized for several decades that chronic phencyclidine abuse may result in persistent psychosis, negative symptoms, thought disorder, and cognitive deficits (Javitt and Zukin 1991) and that acute administration exacerbates symptoms in patients with schizophrenia (Itil et al. 1967). In more recent placebo-controlled trials in which the less-potent NMDA antagonist ketamine was administered intravenously, healthy subjects demonstrated transient, mild psychotic symptoms, negative symptoms, and cognitive deficits that mimicked schizophrenia (Krystal et al. 1994). When administered to nonpsychotic patients with schizophrenia, ketamine produces transient exacerbations of psychotic symptoms that are attenuated by clozapine (Malhotra et al. 1997a) but not by haloperidol (Lahti et al. 1995).

Jentsch and Roth (1999) have argued that chronic administration of NMDA receptor antagonists provides a better model for schizophrenia than does single-dose administration. Prolonged exposure to phencyclidine in substance abusers has been associated with a chronic, severe psychotic illness indistinguishable from schizophrenia (Javitt and Zukin 1991; Jentsch and Roth 1999). Monkeys administered phencyclidine daily for 2 weeks exhibited deficits of working memory that persisted after the drug was discontinued (Jentsch and Roth 1999). Finally, a classical hypofrontal presentation has been observed in chronic phencyclidine-abusing patients (Hertzman et al. 1990).

Interactions Between Dopamine and Glutamate Systems

Phencyclidine acutely increases dopamine concentrations in prefrontal cortex and subcortical structures (Deutch et al. 1987). Chronic administration results in decreased tonic and phasic dopamine release in the prefrontal cortex (Jentsch et al. 1997) and persistent elevation of dopamine release in mesolimbic pathways, particularly the nucleus accumbens (Deutch et al. 1987). Medial prefrontal dopamine utilization (ratio of 3,4-dihydroxyphenylacetic acid [DOPAC, the major metabolite of dopamine] to dopamine) is reduced by as much as 75% in rats after repeated exposure to phencyclidine (Jentsch et al. 1997). The mechanisms by which NMDA antagonists alter dopamine release remain unclear. The initial increase in dopamine release may be mediated by blockade of NMDA receptors on inhibitory GABAergic interneurons, which secondarily disinhibits glutamatergic transmission via non-NMDA receptors (Grunze et al. 1996). Moghaddam and colleagues (1997) reported that the ketamine-induced increase in prefrontal cortical dopamine release and impaired performance on a memory task observed in rats could be ameliorated by LY293558, a KA/AMPA receptor blocker. In contrast, administration of a metabotropic glutamate receptor agonist blocked phencyclidine-induced glutamate release without affecting dopamine release (Moghaddam and Adams 1998).

In addition, NMDA receptor antagonists may disrupt phasic dopamine release via direct effects on NMDA receptors, which modulate mesocortical dopaminergic neurons of the ventral tegmental area. In a series of studies, Svensson and colleagues (1995) examined characteristics of dopamine neuronal firing using pharmacological probes and single-cell recordings from ventral tegmental dopamine neurons in rats. In this model, administration of NMDA antagonists acutely increased the firing rate but decreased the variability of firing, thereby impairing the signal-to-noise ratio. Burst firing was increased in ventral tegmental dopamine neuron cells projecting to limbic regions and was decreased in cells projecting to the prefrontal cortex. Increased mesolimbic dopamine activity associated with long-term administration of phencyclidine produces sensitization to the behavioral effects of NMDA antagonists (phencyclidine, ketamine, and MK801) (Xu and Domino 1994), dopamine agonists, and stress (Jentsch et al. 1998). Subchronic administration of phencyclidine also leads to an increased mesolimbic dopamine response to haloperidol (Jentsch et al. 1998). These findings emphasize the reciprocal modulation of glutamate and dopamine systems and are consistent with the "sensitization model" of schizophrenia (Lieberman et al. 1997).

Psychopharmacology

Current pharmacological treatments for schizophrenia have in common dopamine D_2 receptor antagonism. Relatively selective D_2 antagonists, such as haloperidol, are moderately effective for psychotic symptoms in approximately 70% of patients. Although these drugs may produce modest improvement in negative symptoms, primary negative symptoms are generally unresponsive to D_2 blockade (Goff and Evins 1998). Cognitive deficits also exhibit minimal or no response to conventional antipsychotics (Goldberg and Weinberger 1996). The link between dopamine D_2 receptor blockade and antipsychotic efficacy is strengthened by the highly significant correlation between D_2 receptor affinity and clinical potency of the conventional antipsychotic agents (Creese et al. 1976). Similarly, striatal D_2 receptor occupancy of 65% or greater has been associated with clinical response in vivo using PET ligand-binding studies, and extrapyramidal side effects are typically observed with occupancy greater than 80% (Farde et al. 1992).

Several issues arise concerning mechanisms of action of conventional agents. It is not clear why some patients do not respond to this pharmacological approach. Similarly, the relative lack of responsiveness of negative symptoms and cognitive deficits suggests that dopamine dysregulation is not a primary defect responsible for the full syndrome of schizophrenia. Finally, and possibly most intriguing, it has been observed that several weeks of antipsychotic treatment may be required before full antipsychotic effects are apparent. Because maximal dopamine receptor blockade is achieved within hours of a single dose, this delay suggests that secondary effects occurring "downstream" may be the proximal cause of antipsychotic effects.

Initially, dopamine antagonists increase firing rates of dopamine neurons in the substantia nigra (A9) and ventral tegmental area (A10), presumably acting via presynaptic D_2 autoreceptors (Bunney and Grace 1978). Clinical studies have recorded a corresponding increase in dopamine metabolites at day 4 in CSF and serum; this rise in homovanillic acid (HVA) has correlated significantly with good clinical response in some studies (Pickar 1988). Two to four weeks after initiation of treatment with dopamine antagonists, a substantial proportion of dopamine neurons become electrically silent (Bunney and Grace 1978). This "depolarization blockade" of A9 neurons may mediate extrapyramidal symptoms, and depolarization blockade of mesolimbic A10 neurons may play a role in antipsychotic efficacy. In addition to altering firing patterns of dopamine neurons, subchronic treatment with D_2 receptor antagonists increases postsynaptic D_2 receptor density, which is associated with behavioral "supersensitivity" to dopamine agonists. Recent studies have also demonstrated that subchronic treatment significantly alters the subunit composition of glutamatergic receptors (Fitzgerald et al. 1995). These alterations may represent a change in the pharmacodynamic properties of glutamate receptors on pyramidal neurons and inhibitory interneurons that differs between conventional and atypical agents.

The discovery and characterization of clozapine have contributed to an expanded focus beyond the relatively narrow emphasis on dopamine receptor dysfunction as a putative etiologic mechanism underlying schizophrenia. Clozapine differs from classical dopamine antagonists in possessing greater efficacy for psychotic and negative symptoms while producing few or no neurological side effects (Kane et al. 1988). Clozapine was found to have superior antipsychotic efficacy at dosages producing only 20%–40% D_2 receptor occupancy (Farde et al. 1989). Clozapine also acts at dopamine D_1, D_3, and D_4 receptors, as well as at serotonin 5-HT_2, 5-HT_6, and 5-HT_7 receptors, α-adrenergic receptors, histaminic receptors, and muscarinic receptors (Arnt and Skarsfeldt 1998). Interestingly, preliminary studies suggest that clozapine, unlike conventional agents, blocks ketamine-induced exacerbation of psychotic symptoms mediated by blockade of the glutamatergic NMDA receptor complex (Malhotra et al. 1997a).

The contribution of the different dopamine receptor subtypes to the unique therapeutic advantages of clozapine remains unclear. Although initial reports of clozapine's high affinity for D_4 receptors created considerable enthusiasm, this finding was not replicated (Roth et al. 1995), and preliminary studies of therapeutic agents with selective D_4 antagonism have been disappointing. Treatment with selective D_1 antagonists has similarly been disappointing (Karlsson et al. 1995). The relative importance of 5-HT_{2A} blockade versus D_2 blockade has been shown by these agents to reduce extrapyramidal side effects and to contribute to increased efficacy for negative symptoms (Duinkerke et al. 1993). This combination of relatively higher 5-HT_{2A} over D_2 affinity has been the cornerstone for development of the family of atypical antipsychotic agents that have followed clozapine. In preliminary studies, the addition of idazoxan, an α_2-adrenergic antagonist, to a conventional antipsychotic regimen improved psychotic symptoms (Litman et al. 1996). Several studies have also demonstrated that addition of agonists (glycine, D-cycloserine, and D-serine) at the glutamatergic NMDA receptor complex improve negative symptoms and cognitive deficits (Goff et al. 2001). Cognitive deficits of schizophrenia have remained resistant to pharmacological intervention, although recent preliminary work with an AMPA receptor–positive modulator, or "Ampakine," is promising (Goff et al. 1999).

Conclusions

Pharmacological probes have identified dopamine agonists and glutamatergic NMDA receptor antagonists as models for schizophrenia. Psychotic symptoms produced by amphetamine are blocked by D_2 antagonist treatment, whereas psychotic symptoms produced by ketamine, an NMDA antagonist, are not. Negative symptoms have been associated with decreased activity of prefrontal D_1 receptors and with

NMDA antagonism. Only NMDA antagonists produce cognitive deficits characteristic of schizophrenia. Therapeutic agents that block D_2 receptors typically produce antipsychotic effects after a delay of 2–4 weeks. This suggests that secondary effects, such as depolarization blockade of A10 ventral tegmental dopamine neurons or pharmacodynamic alterations in glutamatergic receptor subunit composition, may play a more proximal role in antipsychotic effects. Addition of 5-HT_{2A} antagonists and NMDA receptor agonists to D_2 blockade improve negative symptoms. The locations of 5-HT_{2A} and NMDA receptors responsible for these therapeutic effects remain unclear and could involve direct modulation of ventral tegmental dopamine neuronal firing or alterations in the sensitivity of inhibitory GABAergic interneurons, which determine cortical pyramidal cell excitability.

The neuropathology of schizophrenia remains elusive. However, postmortem and neuroimaging studies have provided evidence for the involvement of several neural networks in schizophrenia. Impairments in the dorsolateral prefrontal cortex, the thalamus, and the hippocampal formation appear consistently. Abnormalities in these structures might explain some of the diagnostic features of schizophrenia as well as the cognitive deficits often seen in the illness (e.g., memory impairment, attentional deficits, language disturbance).

References

Akbarian S, Bunney WE Jr, Potkin SG, et al: Altered distribution of nicotinamide-adenine dinucleotide phosphate-diaphorase cells in frontal lobe of schizophrenics implies disturbances of cortical development. Arch Gen Psychiatry 50:169–177, 1993

Akbarian S, Kim JJ, Potkin SG, et al: Gene expression for glutamic acid decarboxylase is reduced without loss of neurons in prefrontal cortex of schizophrenics. Arch Gen Psychiatry 52:258–266, 1995

Alpert M: The signs and symptoms of schizophrenia. Compr Psychiatry 26:103–112, 1985

American Psychiatric Association: Diagnostic and Statistical Manual of Mental Disorders, 4th Edition, Text Revision. Washington, DC, American Psychiatric Association, 2000

Andreasen NC: Understanding schizophrenia: a silent spring? Am J Psychiatry 155:1657–1659, 1998

Andreasen NC, Rezai K, Alliger R, et al: Hypofrontality in neuroleptic-naive patients and in patients with chronic schizophrenia: assessment with xenon 133 single-photon emission computed tomography and the Tower of London. Arch Gen Psychiatry 49:943–958, 1992

Andreasen NC, Arndt S, Swayze VN, et al: Thalamic abnormalities in schizophrenia visualized through magnetic resonance image averaging. Science 266:294–298, 1994

Angrist B, Lee HK: The antagonism of amphetamine-induced symptomatology by a neuroleptic. Am J Psychiatry 131:817–819, 1974

Angrist B, Peselow E, Rubinstein M, et al: Partial improvement in negative schizophrenic symptoms after amphetamine. Psychopharmacology (Berl) 78:128–130, 1982

Arnold SE, Hyman BT, Van Hoesen GW, et al: Some cytoarchitectural abnormalities of the entorhinal cortex in schizophrenia. Arch Gen Psychiatry 48:625–632, 1991

Arnt J, Skarsfeldt T: Do novel antipsychotics have similar pharmacological characteristics? A review of evidence. Neuropsychopharmacology 18:63–101, 1998

Beckmann H, Lauer M: The human striatum in schizophrenia, II: increased number of striatal neurons in schizophrenics. Psychiatry Res 68:99–109, 1997

Bell DS: The experimental reproduction of amphetamine psychosis. Arch Gen Psychiatry 29:35–40, 1973

Benes FM, Khan Y, Vincent SL, et al: Differences in the subregional and cellular distribution of GABAA receptor binding in the hippocampal formation of schizophrenic brain. Synapse 22:338–349, 1996a

Benes FM, Vincent SL, Marie A, et al: Up-regulation of GABAA receptor binding on neurons of the prefrontal cortex in schizophrenic subjects. Neuroscience 75:1021–1031, 1996b

Benes FM, Kwok EW, Vincent SL, et al: A reduction of nonpyramidal cells in sector CA2 of schizophrenics and manic depressives. Biol Psychiatry 44:88–97, 1998

Berrios GE: Positive and negative symptoms and Jackson: a conceptual history. Arch Gen Psychiatry 42:95–97, 1985

Bertolino A, Knable MB, Saunders RC, et al: The relationship between dorsolateral prefrontal N-acetylaspartate measures and striatal dopamine activity in schizophrenia. Biol Psychiatry 45:660–667, 1999

Bowers MB: Central dopamine turnover in schizophrenic syndromes. Arch Gen Psychiatry 31:50–54, 1974

Breier A, Su TP, Saunders R, et al: Schizophrenia is associated with elevated amphetamine-induced synaptic dopamine concentrations: evidence from a novel positron emission tomography method. Proc Natl Acad Sci U S A 94:2569–2574, 1997

Buchanan RW, Breier A, Kirkpatrick B, et al: Structural abnormalities in deficit and nondeficit schizophrenia. Am J Psychiatry 150:59–65, 1993

Buchanan RW, Strauss ME, Breier A, et al: Attentional impairments in deficit and nondeficit forms of schizophrenia. Am J Psychiatry 154:363–370, 1997

Bunney BS, Grace AA: Acute and chronic haloperidol treatment: comparison of effects on nigral dopamine cell activity. Life Sci 23:1715–1728, 1978

Callicott JH, Egan MF, Bertolino A, et al: Hippocampal N-acetyl aspartate in unaffected siblings of patients with schizophrenia: a possible intermediate neurobiological phenotype. Biol Psychiatry 44:941–950, 1998

Carpenter WT Jr, Buchanan RW, Kirkpatrick B, et al: Strong inference, theory testing, and the neuroanatomy of schizophrenia. Arch Gen Psychiatry 50: 825–831, 1993

Chakos MH, Lieberman JA, Bilder RM, et al: Increase in caudate nuclei volumes of first-episode schizophrenic patients taking antipsychotic drugs. Am J Psychiatry 151:1430–1436, 1994

Creese I, Burt DR, Snyder SH: Dopamine receptor binding predicts clinical and pharmacological potencies of antischizophrenic drugs. Science 192:481–483, 1976

Crow TJ: The continuum of psychosis and its implication for the structure of the gene. Br J Psychiatry 149:419–429, 1986

Csernansky JG, Joshi S, Wang L, et al: Hippocampal morphometry in schizophrenia by high dimensional brain mapping. Proc Natl Acad Sci U S A 95: 11406–11411, 1998

Danos P, Baumann B, Bernstein HG, et al: Schizophrenia and anteroventral thalamic nucleus: selective decrease of parvalbumin-immunoreactive thalamocortical projection neurons. Psychiatry Res 82:1–10, 1998

Davis KL, Kahn RS, Ko G, et al: Dopamine in schizophrenia: a review and reconceptualization. Am J Psychiatry 148:1474–1486, 1991

DeLisi LE, Buchsbaum MS, Holcomb HH, et al: Increased temporal lobe glucose use in chronic schizophrenic patients. Biol Psychiatry 25:835–851, 1989

Deutch AY, Tam S-Y, Freeman AS, et al: Mesolimbic and mesocortical dopamine activation induced by phencyclidine: contrasting pattern to striatal response. Eur J Pharmacol 134:257–264, 1987

Duinkerke SJ, Botter PA, Jansen AAI, et al: Ritanserin, a selective 5HT2/1c antagonist, and negative symptoms in schizophrenia: a placebo-controlled double blind trial. Br J Psychiatry 163:451–455, 1993

Eastwood SL, Harrison PJ: Decreased synaptophysin in the medial temporal lobe in schizophrenia demonstrated using immunoautoradiography. Neuroscience 69:339–343, 1995

Eastwood SL, McDonald B, Burnet PWJ, et al: Decreased expression of mRNAs encoding non-NMDA glutamate receptors GluR1 and GluR2 in medial temporal lobe neurons in schizophrenia. Brain Res Mol Brain Res 29:211–223, 1995

Ellinwood EJ: Amphetamine psychosis, I: description of the individuals and process. J Nerv Ment Dis 144:273–283, 1967

Farde L, Wiesel FA, Nordstrom AL, et al: D1- and D2-dopamine receptor occupancy during treatment with conventional and atypical neuroleptics. Psychopharmacology (Berl) 99 (suppl):S28–S31, 1989

Farde L, Nordstrom AL, Wiesel FA, et al: Positron emission tomographic analysis of central D1 and D2 dopamine receptor occupancy in patients treated with classical neuroleptics and clozapine: relation to extrapyramidal side effects. Arch Gen Psychiatry 49:538–544, 1992

Fenton WS, McGlashan TH: Natural history of schizophrenia subtypes, I: longitudinal study of paranoid, hebephrenic, and undifferentiated schizophrenia. Arch Gen Psychiatry 48:969–977, 1991

Fitzgerald LW, Deutch AY, Gasic G, et al: Regulation of cortical and subcortical glutamate receptor subunit expression by antipsychotic drugs. J Neurosci 15:2453–2461, 1995

Garey LJ, Ong WY, Patel TS, et al: Reduced dendritic spine density on cerebral cortical pyramidal neurons in schizophrenia. J Neurol Neurosurg Psychiatry 65:446–453, 1998

Goff DC, Coyle JT: The emerging role of glutamate in the pathophysiology and treatment of schizophrenia. Am J Psychiatry 158:1367–1377, 2001

Goff DC, Evins AE: Negative symptoms in schizophrenia: neurobiological models and treatment response. Harv Rev Psychiatry 6:59–77, 1998

Goff DC, Wine L: Glutamate in schizophrenia: clinical and research implications. Schizophr Res 27:157–168, 1997

Goff DC, Bagnell AL, Perlis RH: Glutamatergic augmentation strategies for cognitive impairment in schizophrenia. Psychiatric Annals 29:649–654, 1999

Goldberg TE, Weinberger DR: Effects of neuroleptic medications on the cognition of patients with schizophrenia: a review of recent studies. J Clin Psychiatry 57 (suppl 9):62–65, 1996

Goldman-Rakic PS: Circuitry of the prefrontal cortex and the regulation of behavior by representational knowledge, in Handbook of Physiology. Edited by Plum F, Mountcastle V. Bethesda, MD, American Physiological Society, 1987, pp 373–417

Goldman-Rakic PS: The cortical dopamine system: role in memory and cognition. Adv Pharmacol 42:707–711, 1998

Grace AA: Phasic versus tonic dopamine release and the modulation of dopamine system responsivity: a hypothesis for the etiology of schizophrenia. Neuroscience 41:1–24, 1991

Greden JF, Tandon R: Negative Schizophrenic Symptoms: Pathophysiology and Implications. Washington, DC, American Psychiatric Press, 1991

Grunze HCR, Rainnie DG, Hasselmo ME, et al: NMDA-dependent modulation of CA1 local circuit inhibition. J Neurosci 16:2034–2043, 1996

Gur RE: Functional brain imaging studies in schizophrenia, in Psychopharmacology: The Fourth Generation of Progress. Edited by Bloom FE, Kupfer D. New York, Lippincott-Raven, 1995, pp 1185–1192

Gur RE, Skolnick BE, Gur RC, et al: Brain function in psychiatric disorders, I: regional cerebral blood flow in medicated schizophrenics. Arch Gen Psychiatry 40:1250–1254, 1983

Gur RE, Resnick SM, Alavi A, et al: Regional brain function in schizophrenia, I: a positron emission tomography study. Arch Gen Psychiatry 44:119–125, 1987

Gurevich EV, Bordelon Y, Shapiro RM, et al: Mesolimbic dopamine D3 receptors and use of antipsychotics in patients with schizophrenia: a postmortem study. Arch Gen Psychiatry 54:225–232, 1997

Hazlett EA, Buchsbaum MS, Byne W, et al: Three-dimensional analysis with MRI and PET of the size, shape, and function of the thalamus in the schizophrenia spectrum. Am J Psychiatry 156:1190–1199, 1999

Heckers S: Neuropathology of schizophrenia: cortex, thalamus, basal ganglia, and neurotransmitter-specific projection systems. Schizophr Bull 23:403–421, 1997

Heckers S, Heinsen H, Geiger B, et al: Hippocampal neuron number in schizophrenia: a stereological study. Arch Gen Psychiatry 48:1002–1008, 1991a

Heckers S, Heinsen H, Heinsen Y, et al: Cortex, white matter, and basal ganglia in schizophrenia: a volumetric postmortem study. Biol Psychiatry 29:556–566, 1991b

Heckers S, Rauch SL, Goff D, et al: Impaired recruitment of the hippocampus during conscious recollection in schizophrenia. Nat Neurosci 1:318–323, 1998

Hertzman M, Reba R, Kotlyarove E: Single photon emission computerized tomography in phencyclidine and related drug abuse. Am J Psychiatry 147:255–256, 1990

Hoenig J: Schizophrenia, in A History of Clinical Psychiatry: The Origin and History of Psychiatric Disorders. Edited Berrios GE, Porter R. New York, New York University Press, 1995, pp 336–348

Itil T, Keskiner A, Kiremitci N, et al: Effect of phencyclidine in chronic schizophrenics. Can Psychiatr Assoc J 12:209–212, 1967

Jakab RL, Goldman-Rakic PS: 5-Hydroxytryptamine2A serotonin receptors in the primate cerebral cortex: possible site of action of hallucinogenic and antipsychotic drugs in pyramidal cell apical dendrites. Proc Natl Acad Sci U S A 95:735–740, 1998

Janowsky D, El-Yousef M, Davis J, et al: Provocation of schizophrenic symptoms by intravenous administration of methylphenidate. Arch Gen Psychiatry 28:185–191, 1973

Javitt DC, Zukin SR: Recent advances in the phencyclidine model of schizophrenia. Am J Psychiatry 148:1301–1308, 1991

Jentsch J, Roth R: The neuropsychopharmacology of phencyclidine: from NMDA receptor hypofunction to the dopamine hypothesis of schizophrenia. Neuropsychopharmacology 20:201–225, 1999

Jentsch J, Tran A, Le D, et al: Subchronic phencyclidine administration reduces mesoprefrontal dopamine utilization and impairs prefrontal cortical-dependent cognition in the rat. Neuropsychopharmacology 17:92–99, 1997

Jentsch JD, Taylor JR, Roth RH: Subchronic phencyclidine administration increases mesolimbic dopaminergic system responsivity and augments stress- and psychostimulant-induced hyperlocomotion. Neuropsychopharmacology 19:105–113, 1998

Joyce JN, Shane A, Lexow N, et al: Serotonin uptake sites and serotonin receptors are altered in the limbic system of schizophrenics. Neuropsychopharmacology 8:315–336, 1993

Kalus P, Senitz D, Beckmann H: Cortical layer I changes in schizophrenia: a marker for impaired brain development. J Neural Transm 104:549–559, 1997

Kane J, Honigfeld G, Singer J, et al: Clozapine for the treatment-resistant schizophrenic: a double-blind comparison with chlorpromazine. Arch Gen Psychiatry 45:789–796, 1988

Karlsson P, Smith L, Farde L, et al: Lack of apparent antipsychotic effect of the D1-dopamine receptor antagonist SCH39166 in acutely ill schizophrenic patients. Psychopharmacology (Berl) 121:309–316, 1995

Kawasaki Y, Suzuki M, Maeda Y, et al: Regional cerebral blood flow in patients with schizophrenia. A preliminary report. Eur Arch Psychiatry Clin Neurosci 241:195–200, 1992

Kegeles LS, Humaran TJ, Mann JJ: In vivo neurochemistry of the brain in schizophrenia as revealed by magnetic resonance spectroscopy. Biol Psychiatry 44:382–398, 1998

Kendell RE, Cooper JE, Gourlay AG: Diagnostic criteria of American and British psychiatrists. Arch Gen Psychiatry 25:123–130, 1971

Keshavan MS, Rosenberg D, Sweeney JA, et al: Decreased caudate volume in neuroleptic-naive psychotic patients. Am J Psychiatry 155:774–778, 1998

Knable MB, Hyde TM, Murray AM, et al: A postmortem study of frontal cortical dopamine D1 receptors in schizophrenics, psychiatric controls, and normal controls. Biol Psychiatry 40:1191–1199, 1996

Kraepelin E: Dementia Praecox and Paraphrenia. Edinburgh, Livingstone, 1919

Krystal JH, Karper LP, Seibyl JP, et al: Subanesthetic effects of the noncompetitive NMDA antagonist, ketamine, in humans: psychotomimetic, perceptual, cognitive, and neuroendocrine responses. Arch Gen Psychiatry 51:199–214, 1994

Kung L, Conley R, Chute DJ, et al: Synaptic changes in the striatum of schizophrenic cases: a controlled postmortem ultrastructural study. Synapse 28: 125–139, 1998

Lahti AC, Koffel B, LaPorte D, et al: Subanesthetic doses of ketamine stimulate psychosis in schizophrenia. Neuropsychopharmacology 13:9–19, 1995

Laruelle M, Abi-Dargham A, van Dyck CH, et al: Single photon emission computerized tomography imaging of amphetamine-induced dopamine release in drug-free schizophrenic subjects. Proc Natl Acad Sci U S A 93:9235–9240, 1996

Leonhard K: Aufteilung der endogenen Psychosen und ihre differenzierte Ätiologie. Stuttgart, Georg Thieme Verlag, 1995

Lewis R, Kapur S, Jones C, et al: Serotonin 5-HT2 receptors in schizophrenia: a PET study using [18F]setoperone in neuroleptic-naive patients and normal subjects. Am J Psychiatry 156:72–78, 1999

Liddle PF, Friston KJ, Frith CD, et al: Patterns of cerebral blood flow in schizophrenia. Br J Psychiatry 160:179–186, 1992

Lidow MS, Williams GV, Goldman-Rakic PS: The cerebral cortex: a case for a common site of action of antipsychotics. Trends Pharmacol Sci 19:136–140, 1998

Lidsky TI: Neuropsychiatric implications of basal ganglia dysfunction. Biol Psychiatry 41:383–385, 1997

Lieberman JA, Koreen AR: Neurochemistry and neuroendocrinology of schizophrenia: a selective review. Schizophr Bull 19:371–429, 1993

Lieberman JA, Kane JM, Gadaleta D, et al: Methylphenidate challenge as a predictor of relapse in schizophrenia. Am J Psychiatry 141:633–638, 1984

Lieberman JA, Sheitman BB, Kinon BJ: Neurochemical sensitization in the pathophysiology of schizophrenia: deficits and dysfunction in neuronal regulation and plasticity. Neuropsychopharmacology 17:205–229, 1997

Litman RE, Su T-P, Potter WZ, et al: Idazozan and response to typical neuroleptics in treatment-resistant schizophrenia. Br J Psychiatry 168:571–579, 1996

Machiyama YL: Chronic methamphetamine intoxication model of schizophrenia in animals. Schizophr Bull 18:107–113, 1992

Malhotra AK, Adler CM, Kennison SD, et al: Clozapine blunts N-methyl-D-aspartate antagonist-induced psychosis: a study with ketamine. Biol Psychiatry 42:664–668, 1997a

Malhotra AK, Pinals DA, Adler CM, et al: Ketamine-induced exacerbation of psychotic symptoms and cognitive impairment in neuroleptic-free schizophrenics. Neuropsychopharmacology 17:141–150, 1997b

Mathew RJ, Duncan GC, Weinman ML, et al: Regional cerebral blood flow in schizophrenia. Arch Gen Psychiatry 39:1121–1124, 1982

McCarley RW, Wible CG, Frumin M, et al: MRI anatomy of schizophrenia. Biol Psychiatry 45:1099–1119, 1999

Moghaddam B, Adams BW: Reversal of phencyclidine effects by a group II metabotropic glutamate receptor agonist. Science 281:1349–1352, 1998

Moghaddam B, Adams B, Verma A, et al: Activation of glutamatergic neurotransmission by ketamine: a novel step in the pathway from NMDA receptor blockade to dopaminergic and cognitive disruptions associated with the prefrontal cortex. J Neurosci 17:2921–2927, 1997

Mrzljak L, Bergson C, Pappy M, et al: Localization of dopamine D4 receptors in GABAergic neurons of the primate brain. Nature 381:245–248, 1996

Muly EC 3rd, Szigeti K, Goldman-Rakic PS: D1 receptor in interneurons of macaque prefrontal cortex: distribution and subcellular localization. J Neurosci 18:10553–10565, 1998

Okubo Y, Suhara T, Suzuki K, et al: Decreased prefrontal dopamine D1 receptors in schizophrenia revealed by PET. Nature 385:634–636, 1997

Pakkenberg B: Pronounced reduction of total neuron number in mediodorsal thalamic nucleus and nucleus accumbens in schizophrenics. Arch Gen Psychiatry 47:1023–1028, 1990

Palha AP, Esteves MF: The origin of dementia praecox. Schizophr Res 28:99–103, 1997

Papez JW: A proposed mechanism of emotion. Arch Neurol Psychiatry 38:725–743, 1937

Perrone-Bizzozero NI, Sower AC, Bird ED, et al: Levels of the growth-associated protein GAP-43 are selectively increased in association cortices in schizophrenia. Proc Natl Acad Sci U S A 93:14182–14187, 1996

Pickar D: Perspectives on a time-dependent model of neuroleptic action. Schizophr Bull 14:255–268, 1988

Port RL, Sample JA, Seybold KS: Partial hippocampal pyramidal cell loss alters behavior in rats: implications for an animal model of schizophrenia. Brain Res Bull 26:993–996, 1991

Portas CM, Goldstein JM, Shenton ME, et al: Volumetric evaluation of the thalamus in schizophrenic male patients using magnetic resonance imaging. Biol Psychiatry 43:649–659, 1998

Pycock CJ, Kerwin RW, Carter CJ: Effect of lesion of cortical dopamine terminals on sub-cortical dopamine receptors in rats. Nature 286:74–77, 1980

Roth BL, Tandra S, Burgess LH, et al: D4 dopamine receptor binding affinity does not distinguish between typical and atypical antipsychotic drugs. Psychopharmacology (Berl) 120:365–368, 1995

Sartorius N, Üstün, BAK, Cooper JE, et al: Progress towards achieving a common language in psychiatry, II: results from the international field trials of the ICD-10 diagnostic criteria for research for mental and behavioral disorders. Am J Psychiatry 152:1427–1437, 1995

Sato M: Acute exacerbation of methamphetamine psychosis and lasting dopaminergic supersensitivity: a clinical survey. Psychopharmacol Bull 22:751–756, 1986

Saunders RC, Kolachana BS, Bachevalier J, et al: Neonatal lesions of the medial temporal lobe disrupt prefrontal cortical regulation of striatal dopamine. Nature 393:169–171, 1998

Scheibel AB: The thalamus and neuropsychiatric illness. J Neuropsychiatry Clin Neurosci 9:342–353, 1997

Schmajuk NA: Animal models for schizophrenia: the hippocampally lesioned animal. Schizophr Bull 13:317–327, 1987

Schneider K: Clinical Psychopathology. New York, Grune & Stratton, 1959

Sedvall G, Farde L: Chemical brain anatomy in schizophrenia. Lancet 346:743–749, 1995

Selemon LD, Rajkowska G, Goldman-Rakic PS: Abnormally high neuronal density in.the schizophrenic cortex: a morphometric analysis of prefrontal area 9 and occipital area 17. Arch Gen Psychiatry 52:805–818, 1995

Silbersweig DA, Stern E, Frith C, et al: A functional neuroanatomy of hallucinations in schizophrenia. Nature 378:176–179, 1995

Simpson MD, Slater P, Deakin JF, et al: Reduced GABA uptake sites in the temporal lobe in schizophrenia. Neurosci Lett 107:211–215, 1989

Southard EE: On the topographical distribution of cortex lesions and anomalies in dementia praecox, with some account of their functional significance. American Journal of Insanity 71:383–403, 1914

Svensson TH, Mathe JM, Andersson JL, et al: Mode of action of atypical neuroleptics in relation to the phencyclidine model of schizophrenia: role of 5-HT2 receptor and alpha1-adrenoreceptor antagonism. J Clin Psychopharmacol 15 (1 suppl 1):11S–18S, 1995

Tamminga CA, Thaker GK, Buchanan R, et al: Limbic system abnormalities identified in schizophrenia using positron emission tomography with fluorodeoxyglucose and neocortical alterations with deficit syndrome. Arch Gen Psychiatry 49:522–530, 1992

Van Hoesen GW: The parahippocampal gyrus: new observations regarding its cortical connections in the monkey. Trends Neurosci 5:345–350, 1982

Van Kammen DP, Boronow JJ: Dextro-amphetamine diminishes negative symptoms in schizophrenia. Int Clin Psychopharmacol 3:111–121, 1988

Velakoulis D, Pantelis C, McGorry PD, et al: Hippocampal volume in first-episode psychoses and chronic schizophrenia: a high-resolution magnetic resonance imaging study. Arch Gen Psychiatry 56:133–141, 1999

Volkow ND, Wolf AP, Van Gelder P, et al: Phenomenological correlates of metabolic activity in 18 patients with chronic schizophrenia. Am J Psychiatry 144:151–158, 1987

Weinberger DR, Berman KF, Zec RF: Physiologic dysfunction of dorsolateral prefrontal cortex in schizophrenia, I: regional cerebral blood flow evidence [see comments]. Arch Gen Psychiatry 43:114–124, 1986

Weinberger DR, Berman KF, Suddath R, et al: Evidence of dysfunction of a prefrontal-limbic network in schizophrenia: a magnetic resonance imaging and regional cerebral blood flow study of discordant monzygotic twins. Am J Psychiatry 149:890–897, 1992

Woo TU, Whitehead RE, Melchitzky DS, et al: A subclass of prefrontal gamma-aminobutyric acid axon terminals are selectively altered in schizophrenia. Proc Natl Acad Sci U S A 95:5341–5346, 1998

Xu X, Domino EF: Phencyclidine-induced behavioral sensitization. Pharmacol Biochem Behav 47:603–608, 1994

CHAPTER 4

Neural Circuitry and Signaling in Addiction

Ronald P. Hammer Jr., Ph.D.

Addiction medicine has recently witnessed a paradigm shift that has introduced neuroscience and molecular neurobiology to the field. Even the definition of addiction has changed in the past 20 years; addiction was previously defined as habituation, or reduced responsiveness, to a practice considered harmful (Stedman 1977). It is now viewed as habitual psychological and physiological dependence on a substance or practice that is beyond voluntary control (Dirckx 1997). The latter definition implies the development of involuntary compulsive behaviors related to a neurobiological etiology. Rather than viewing addiction as a deliberate selection of behavior, the process and outcome of addiction should be viewed as a *disease.* The individual's predisposition to acquire self-administration of abused substances, the magnitude of initial biological responses, and the adaptive alterations of cellular transduction systems within critical neural pathways each contribute to the severity of addiction. The implication is that effective therapies must alter both the biological substrates for addiction and the ongoing social and environmental factors that influence it. As stated in the title of a recent review article, "Addiction is a brain disease, and it matters" (Leshner 1997).

Addiction is often, although not always, associated with psychoactive substances such as drugs or alcohol. Most of our knowledge about the biological substrates for addiction is derived from the effects of these substances. Therefore, the following discussion will relate mostly to the consequences of psychoactive substance use. It should be noted that the current definition of addiction (above) includes compulsive

This work was supported by U.S Public Health Service Awards DA09822 and MH60251.

practices (e.g., eating, sex, Internet browsing) that might also involve the same brain circuits and signaling pathways.

Clinical Presentation

Classification of substance use disorders can assist in diagnosis and recognition of the behavioral and physiological symptoms. Criteria for the diagnosis of medical disorders associated with substance use in DSM-IV-TR (American Psychiatric Association 2000) differentiate substance abuse from dependence, both of which are associated with a variety of psychoactive substances. Substance abuse is defined as a maladaptive pattern of substance use that causes significant impairment (e.g., social or occupational) or physical hazard (e.g., driving while intoxicated). Substance dependence adds the presence of *uncontrollable* substance use and persistent desire for substances having adverse consequences, and includes the development of tolerance and/or withdrawal symptoms. Thus, dependence may lead to greater intake as the same stimulus produces lesser response upon repeated exposure. Some substances, notably psychostimulants, may produce a progressive enhancement of motor or other responses known as *sensitization,* even though drug intake might still increase due to the concurrent development of tolerance to the subjective effects. In a dependent individual, abrupt cessation of substance use can produce a physiological and/or behavioral withdrawal syndrome whose symptoms and severity depend on the particular substance(s) used. The enduring nature of symptoms and the vulnerability to repeated relapse associated with substance dependence, even in the absence of continued use, suggests that persistent changes of brain structure and function underlie these symptoms. Such alterations might give rise to the maladaptive and uncontrollable pattern of substance use characteristic of abuse or dependence.

Neural Circuitry

Most substances that are reinforcing (i.e., promote self-administration or reward) are known to increase the level of dopamine in the nucleus accumbens (NAc). The source of this dopamine is a collection of mesocorticolimbic neurons located in the floor of the midbrain, or the ventral tegmental area (VTA), that project rostrally through the medial forebrain bundle to supply the NAc, amygdala, and prefrontal cortical regions in mammalian brains (*bold lines* in Figure 4–1). Electrical stimulation of the VTA or the medial forebrain bundle is reinforcing and increases dopamine release in the NAc (Fiorino et al. 1993). The NAc also receives substantial input from the prefrontal cortex, hippocampus, and amygdala, each of which contributes axonal fibers containing the excitatory neurotransmitter glutamate (*dotted lines* in Figure 4–1; Wright and Groenewegen 1995). Additional neurotransmitters, including norepinephrine and serotonin, are supplied by afferent input from brain-stem neurons, and endogenous opioid peptides, acetylcholine, and γ-aminobutyric acid (GABA) are derived from intrinsic striatal neurons. Thus, dopamine release or response could be mediated by pharmacological or environmental alteration of a rich array of neurotransmitters in the NAc.

Extrinsic projection neurons in the NAc are components of long feedback loops that influence either the cortex (via pallidothalamic relay) or the VTA. All NAc projection neurons contain the inhibitory neurotransmitter GABA and are dopaminoceptive. Those neurons that provide reciprocal innervation to the VTA, similar to the direct-projection neurons of the dorsal striatum, contain the neuropeptides dynorphin and substance P (*dashed lines* in Figure 4–1) and predominantly express dopamine D_1-like receptors (Le Moine and Bloch 1995) and adenosine A_1 receptors (Ferre et al. 1996). Those neurons that predominantly express D_1-like receptors innervate both the ventral pallidum (VP) and the VTA. Another population of NAc projection neurons innervate the ventral pallidum, contain the neuropeptide enkephalin (*long-dashed line* in Figure 4–1), and predominantly express dopamine D_2-like receptors and adenosine A_{2A} receptors (Gerfen et al. 1995). Ventral pallidal neurons innervate the mediodorsal thalamic nucleus, which sends projections to cortical regions (*nonbold solid lines* in Figure 4–1), thereby completing the cortico-striato-pallido-thalamo-cortical circuit. Thus, two distinct phenotypes of NAc projection neurons exist, each with its own neurochemical, pharmacological, and neuroanatomic characteristics.

The heterogeneous characteristics of NAc neurons are further complicated by regional and cellular divisions within the NAc. The NAc can be separated into a medial shell region associated with limbic functions and a lateral core region associated with motor function (Voorn et al. 1996). The further segregation of neurochemical compartments—called *patch* (or *striosome*) and *matrix*—in the dorsal striatum appears to be quite complex in the NAc (Jongen-Relo et al. 1993). Furthermore, the NAc shell has been found to exhibit phenotypic similarity to the amygdala, extending along a continuum through the basal forebrain that has been termed the *extended amygdala.* This entire region responds to reinforcing substances and may serve as a powerful substrate for behavioral changes occurring during dependence and withdrawal (Koob 1999).

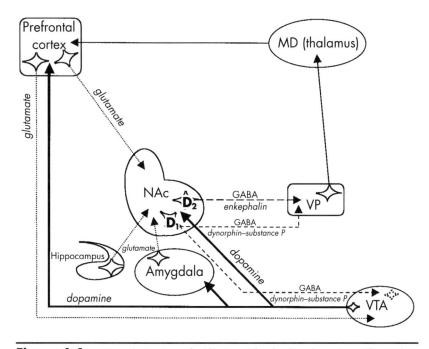

Figure 4–1.   *Neural circuitry of addiction. Like the dorsal striatum, the nucleus accumbens (NAc) in the ventral striatum receives innervation from the midbrain and cortex. Cortical input from prefrontal neurons, as well as from the amygdala and hippocampus, is glutamatergic* **(dotted lines)**. *Mesocorticolimbic dopamine originates from neurons in the ventral tegmental area (VTA), which innervate the NAc, amygdala, and various regions of prefrontal cortex* **(bold lines)**. *Dopamine modulates the activity of NAc neurons by binding to D_1- or D_2-like receptors, which are expressed by distinct populations of NAc projection neurons. Those neurons that express predominantly D_1-like receptors innervate both the ventral pallidum (VP) and the VTA* **(dashed lines)**, *whereas neurons expressing predominantly D_2-like receptors innervate the VP* **(long-dashed line)**. *Both types of NAc projection neurons contain γ-aminobutyric acid (GABA), but D_2-like receptor–containing cells also contain enkephalin and D_1-like receptor–containing cells also contain substance P and dynorphin. VP neurons (which also receive VTA dopamine innervation) innervate the mediodorsal nucleus (MD) of the thalamus, which in turn projects to the prefrontal cortex to complete this limbic cortico-striato-pallido-thalamo-cortical loop. NAc neurons are richly innervated by many other neurotransmitters from intrinsic and extrinsic sources. Dopamine modulates the activity of striatal neurons in response to the amount of glutamate in the environs and the state of the neuron. Stimulation of D_1-like receptors increases the excitability of striatal neurons in the presence of glutamate, but inhibits activity in the absence of cortical input. D_2-like receptor stimulation reduces striatal neuron activity.*

Signaling Pathways

Although many neurotransmitters affect NAc neurons, it is generally agreed that dopamine is responsible for the major reinforcing properties of most abused substances. For example, the reinforcing efficacy of intracranial self-stimulation is impaired by pretreatment with pimozide, a dopamine receptor antagonist, and is enhanced by amphetamine, a drug that releases dopamine in the NAc (Gallistel and Karras 1984). Furthermore, the self-administration potency of cocaine-like drugs is correlated with inhibition of the dopamine transporter (Ritz et al. 1987). Many other drugs of abuse also increase extracellular dopamine levels in the NAc either directly by enhancing the activity of VTA dopamine neurons (e.g., opioids) or indirectly by another mechanism (e.g., alcohol, cannabinoids, nicotine). Naturally reinforcing stimuli such as food or sex also increase extracellular NAc dopamine, albeit to a lesser extent and with greater habituation following repeated exposure than do drug stimuli (Di Chiara 1998).

Other neurotransmitters, such as the excitatory amino acid glutamate, also are implicated in the reinforcing effects of abused substances. Glutamate can act at dopamine terminals to release dopamine in the NAc, and abused substances can alter glutamatergic response in dopamine neurons. For example, alcohol selectively inhibits the *N*-methyl-D-aspartate (NMDA) receptor subunit NMDA-R2B. Furthermore, glutamate signaling can adapt with repeated drug exposure, as exemplified by the finding of upregulation of various NMDA and α-amino-3-hydroxy-5-methyl-4-isoxazole-propionic acid (AMPA) receptor subunits in the VTA and NAc in response to repeated cocaine or morphine administration in animals that exhibit behavioral sensitization (Churchill et al. 1999). Finally, recent evidence suggests that stimulation of NAc AMPA receptors enhances the reinforcing effect of cocaine and facilitates reinstatement of cocaine self-administration (Cornish et al. 1999).

Dopamine probably provides complementary modulation of different pathways from the NAc as a result of the apparent segregation of dopamine D_1- and D_2-like receptors on different populations of efferent neurons (see Figure 4–1). These complementary effects may be related to the opposite intracellular responses produced by the signal transduction systems coupled to D_1- and D_2-like receptors. D_1-like receptors are coupled to adenylyl cyclase by a stimulatory heterotrimeric guanosine triphosphate–binding protein (stimulatory G protein, or G_s), invoking cyclic adenosine 3′,5′-monophosphate (cAMP) production following D_1-like receptor stimulation (Figure 4–2, left). In contrast, D_2-like receptors are coupled to adenylyl cyclase by inhibitory G proteins (G_i/G_o), result-

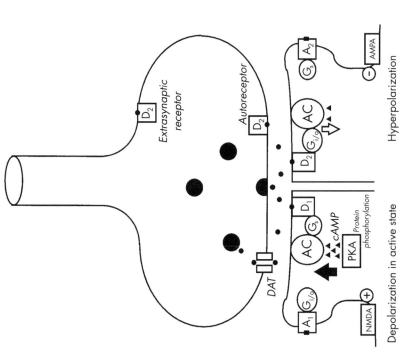

Figure 4–2. *The dopamine synapse. Dopaminergic terminals contain dense core vesicles* **(large solid circles)** *that store and concentrate dopamine through the action of vesicular monoamine transporters. Arrival of an action potential stimulates opening of voltage-gated Ca^{2+} channels and exocytosis of vesicles to release dopamine* **(small solid circles)**. *Released dopamine may bind to presynaptic D_2-like autoreceptors that reduce tyrosine hydroxylase function in terminals, extrasynaptic receptors, or postsynaptic receptors. Most dopamine is removed from the synapse through reuptake into presynaptic terminals by dopamine transporters (DAT). D_2-like postsynaptic receptors* **(lower right)** *are negatively coupled to adenylyl cyclase (AC) by G proteins (G_i/G_o). D_2-like receptor stimulation reduces cAMP* **(solid triangles)**, *attenuates AMPA receptor activity, and opens K^+ channels, leading to neuronal hyperpolarization. D_1-like receptors* **(lower left)** *are positively coupled to AC by a stimulatory G protein (G_s), which increases cAMP upon stimulation. D_1-like receptor activation increases cAMP and activate protein kinase A (PKA) to induce phosphorylation of intracellular proteins. D_1-like receptor activation reduces K^+ and enhances L-type Ca^{2+} channel flux, and potentiates glutamate responses mediated by the NMDA receptor to depolarize neurons. D_1- and D_2-like receptors are expressed in neurons that also contain adenosine A_1 and A_{2A} receptors, respectively. These adenosine receptors are coupled to AC by G_i/G_o and G_s, respectively, which may help to compensate for continued D_1- and D_2-like receptor activity.*

Upon repeated psychostimulant treatment, which increases dopamine level, $G_i/G_o\alpha$ is reduced **(open arrow)**, *which normalizes cAMP level in D_2-like receptor–containing neurons. In contrast, repeated psychostimulant treatment increases AC and PKA* **(filled arrow)**, *leading to enhanced protein phosphorylation, D_1-like receptor supersensitivity, depolarization of D_1-like receptor–containing neurons, and behavioral sensitization.*

$G_i/G_o = G_i/G_o$ proteins; AMPA = α-amino-3-hydroxy-5-methyl-4-isoxalone propionic acid; cAMP = cyclic adenosine 3′,5′-monophosphate; NMDA = N-methyl-D-aspartate.

ing in reduced cAMP following D_2-like receptor stimulation (Figure 4–2, right). An increase in cAMP levels results in activation of protein kinase A (PKA). Activated PKA phosphorylates intracellular proteins, such as transcription factors (e.g., cAMP response element binding protein [CREB]) and DARPP-32 (a potent inhibitor of protein phosphatase found in all D_1-like receptor–containing striatal neurons), as well as volt-age-gated (e.g., Ca^{2+} and K^+ channels) and ligand-gated (e.g., NMDA) ion channels. Dopamine release thus increases the excitability of striatal neurons via D_1-like receptors by reducing K^+ inactivation currents, en-hancing L-type Ca^{2+} channel conductance, and potentiating NMDA re-ceptor–mediated responses (Cepeda and Levine 1998).

The effects of D_1-like dopamine receptor stimulation differ depend-ing on the amount of glutamate present in the microenvironment. D_1 agonists enhance evoked discharge of striatal neurons at relatively de-polarized membrane potentials in response to cortical input, but they inhibit discharge at hyperpolarized membrane potentials in the absence of cortical input—for example, in vitro or anesthetized preparations (Hernández-Lopez et al. 1997). Again in contrast to D_1-like receptors, stimulation of D_2-like receptors attenuates responses mediated by glutamatergic activation of non-NMDA receptors and induces K^+ chan-nel opening (Cepeda and Levine 1998). D_1- and D_2-like receptors also appear to differentially regulate the expression of long-term potentia-tion and depression in striatal neurons following cortical stimulation, suggesting their involvement in controlling the direction of synaptic plasticity (Calabresi et al. 2000). Thus, striatal neuronal responses in-volved in conditioned learning may differ according to the type of do-pamine receptor stimulation. Many of the above discoveries stem from the dorsal striatum; however, the presence of homologous neurochem-ical, pharmacological, and molecular substrates in the NAc suggest that similar mechanisms apply therein.

The divergent effects of dopamine on functional activity of striatal neurons might be due to differing effects of D_1- and D_2-like receptors. These different dopaminoceptive pathways use the same signal trans-duction system (cAMP pathways) to yield complementary responses. Dopamine-induced striatal immediate-early gene expression and co-caine-induced activation of direct striatonigral projection neurons are cAMP-dependent processes that are blocked by D_1-like receptor antag-onists (Chergui et al. 1996; Thomas et al. 1996). Cocaine and amphet-amine induction of immediate-early gene expression is dependent on CREB (Hyman et al. 1995) in direct projection neurons, as is immediate-early gene induction by haloperidol, a D_2-like receptor antagonist (Kon-radi and Heckers 1995), in indirect projection neurons. Immediate-early gene induction occurs similarly in projection neurons of the NAc (Robertson and Jian 1995), where CREB overexpression reduces the reinforcing efficacy of cocaine (Carlezon et al. 1998).

Intracellular Consequences of Drug Exposure

The behavioral consequences of repeated drug exposure appear to be mainly the result of compensatory responses by intracellular transduction systems affecting the number, affinity, or function of available receptors. Regulation of such alterations, however, involves adaptation of receptor–G protein coupling that may produce desensitization and downregulation following exposure to direct or indirect agonists such as opioids or psychostimulants (Nestler and Aghajanian 1997). Short-term changes in response may be produced via phosphorylation of receptors by G protein receptor kinase (GRK) (Pitcher et al. 1998). Following agonist binding and GRK-mediated phosphorylation of activated receptors, binding of β-arrestin protein uncouples receptors from their associated G proteins and initiates the process of sequestration and receptor internalization. This leads to rapid desensitization and ultimately to trafficking of receptors either through recycling to the cell membrane in an active, resensitized state or toward degradation and downregulation of receptor number. Whether this mechanism is involved in the prolonged effects of repeated drug exposure remains unclear. In fact, some opioid drugs of abuse might circumvent this recycling mechanism entirely to produce physiological tolerance. Morphine is a potent activator of μ opioid receptors but induces neither G protein uncoupling nor receptor internalization, whereas methadone and etorphine promote internalization (Whistler et al. 1999). Thus, phosphorylation and endocytosis of activated μ opioid receptors might serve a protective role to reduce the development of tolerance.

Cellular and Molecular Adaptations Caused by Repeated Drug Exposure

Adaptations occurring as a result of repeated drug exposure are dependent on the characteristics of the neuron involved. For example, in the NAc, the D_2-like receptor system becomes subsensitive following repeated cocaine challenge, whereas the D_1-like receptor system becomes supersensitive, exhibiting upregulation of the cAMP pathway. Repeated stimulation of D_2-like receptors decreases expression of the α subunit of the G_i/G_o family of G proteins (Figure 4–2, right; Nestler et al. 1990), which reduces both cocaine and opioid reinforcement (Self et al. 1994). The result is a compensatory reduction of the G_i/G_o-mediated inhibitory influence on adenylyl cyclase to normalize cAMP levels in these neurons. This change could be mediated by a novel class of proteins known as *regulator of G protein signaling* (RGS) proteins, which accelerate intrinsic guanosine triphosphatase (GTPase) activity in α subunits, thereby limiting receptor-effector coupling. RGS9-2 is expressed selectively in neurons of the NAc and striatum and may target $G_i/G_o\alpha$ proteins (Rahman et al. 1999) associated with μ opioid or D_2-like receptors. In contrast, repeated cocaine administration increases adenylyl cyclase and PKA activity in the NAc (Terwilliger et al. 1991) via dopaminergic stimulation of D_1-like receptors (Figure 4–2, left). Enhancement of PKA leads to increased cocaine self-administration and drug tolerance (Self et al. 1998), which may be mediated by increased phosphorylation of CREB. Enhanced CREB activation induces the expression of dynorphin (Carlezon et al. 1998), which stimulates κ opioid receptors in regions containing terminals of NAc projection neurons. Tolerance to the subjective effects of cocaine also occurs in cocaine-dependent human subjects as compared with drug-abstinent individuals who report occasional cocaine use (Mendelson et al. 1998). Similar upregulation of the cAMP pathway is found following chronic alcohol exposure (Ortiz et al. 1995), as well as in rat strains that exhibit greater preference for opioids, cocaine, and alcohol, suggesting that genetic predisposition might enhance tolerance and facilitate dependence (Beitner-Johnson et al. 1991).

Repeated exposure to psychostimulants, opioids, nicotine, and other abused substances also induces accumulation of a unique isoform of the transcription factor ΔFosB in D_1-like receptor–containing neurons of the NAc (Nestler et al. 1999b). This chronic ΔFosB isoform, which can persist for weeks, even without subsequent drug exposure, heterodimerizes with JunD or JunB to form an activator protein (AP) complex. This complex binds to an AP-1 consensus site located in the 5′-promoter region of certain target genes to alter their expression. Chronic overexpression of ΔFosB in the striatum causes an enhanced behavioral response to cocaine that is mediated, at least in part, by induction of the GluR2 subunit of the AMPA receptor in the NAc (Kelz et al. 1999). This effect might underlie the enhancement of cocaine reinforcement by NAc AMPA receptor stimulation in animals trained to self-administer cocaine (Cornish et al. 1999).

The pharmacokinetics of opioids differ from those of cocaine, but the two drugs have similar neuroadaptive responses following chronic exposure. Although opioids directly affect signaling in the NAc, much more is known about their effects in the locus coeruleus (LC) (Nestler et al. 1999a), the major source of forebrain noradrenergic innervation. LC neurons normally fire tonically, but their firing rate increases in response to stressful or noxious stimuli, heightening alertness and stimulating sympathetic activity. Acutely, opioids stimulate the μ receptor to produce G protein–mediated changes in channel function affecting LC neuronal activity (Figure 4–3, left). The ligand-bound μ receptor dissociates the G_i/G_o heterotrimer to which it is coupled into an α subunit bound to GTP and a β-γ subunit. The free β-γ subunit then binds to a G protein–activated, inwardly rectifying K$^+$ (GIRK) channel, causing the channel to open and reducing membrane potential. In addition, the activated G_i/G_oα inhibits adenylyl cyclase, decreasing cAMP and reducing PKA activity. This reduces current flow through a nonspecific cation channel, thereby blocking depolarization. The combined effect of opioids acting acutely at the μ receptor is to inhibit LC neuronal activity.

Opioid use in dependent individuals tends to be chronic and continuous, causing upregulation of the cAMP pathway due to increased levels of adenylyl cyclase and PKA as well as tyrosine hydroxylase in LC neurons (Figure 4–3, right). Sustained inhibition of PKA by chronic opioid treatment leads to a compensatory increase in CREB expression due to autoregulation. The adenylyl cyclase (isoform VII) and tyrosine hydroxylase genes both contain a cAMP response element site in their promoters, so CREB induction increases their transcription. Furthermore, experimental reduction of CREB expression by injection of CREB antisense oligonucleotides into the LC eliminates upregulation of adenylyl cyclase and tyrosine hydroxylase by morphine (Lane-Ladd et al. 1997). Opioid treatment ultimately increases PKA level due to increased stabilization and reduced degradation of PKA subunits. The overall effect of *chronic* opioid cAMP pathway upregulation in the LC is reinstitution of normal GIRK and nonspecific cation channel activity, leading to a recovery of normal firing rate in the presence of sustained opioid stimulation (i.e., while on drugs).

It should be noted that chronic opioid-induced changes in the LC probably do not influence the reinforcing or stimulant properties of opioids, even though they affect the individual's somatic and behavioral state. Nevertheless, μ opioid receptors provide a critical substrate for opioid reinforcement, given that experimental animals lacking the μ receptor exhibit neither reinforcing effects from morphine nor cAMP pathway upregulation following chronic morphine treatment (Matthes et al. 1996). In addition, the CB$_1$ cannabinoid receptor (which binds delta-9-tetrahydrocannabinol [Δ^9-THC], the psychoactive component of marijuana) may be involved in the reinforcing effects of opioids, because deletion of the CB$_1$ receptor prevents morphine self-administration (Ledent et al. 1999). Opioid exposure produces upregulation of the GluR1 subunit of the AMPA receptor in the VTA (Fitzgerald et al. 1996). This effect intensifies both opioid reinforcement and behavioral sensiti-

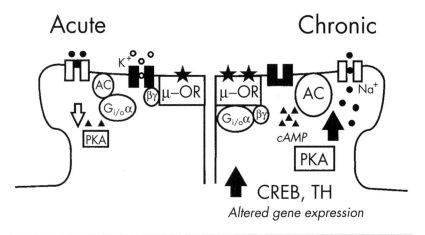

Figure 4–3.   *Opioid effects mediated by the μ-opioid receptor (μ-OR). The μ-OR is coupled to a heterotrimeric G protein of the G_i/G_o family. Acutely (left), exogenous opioids bind to the μ receptor, causing dissociation of the α and β-γ G protein subunits. The β-γ subunit opens an inwardly rectifying channel (solid boxes), allowing K^+ efflux, which reduces the membrane potential. The activated G_i/G_oα inhibits adenylyl cyclase (AC) to reduce cAMP (solid triangles) and PKA activity (open arrow). This reduces conductance in nonspecific cation channels (open boxes), blocking further depolarization. Opioids act acutely to inhibit neuronal activity.*

Chronic opioid binding (right) causes upregulation of the cAMP pathway in neurons of the locus coeruleus. A compensatory induction of CREB expression increases AC transcription, whereas PKA probably increases due to reduced degradation of activated PKA subunits. The expression of various genes that respond to CREB or other phosphoproteins is altered. Overall, the effect of chronic opioid stimulation is recovery of K^+ and cation channel function leading to normalized neuronal firing even in the presence of opioid.

Removal of μ-opioid stimulation in the presence of cAMP pathway upregulation leads to neuronal hyperactivity. Hyperexcitable locus coeruleus neurons enhance noradrenergic tone, stimulate sympathetic activity, and induce anxiety.

PKA = protein kinase A; G_i/G_oα = alpha subunit of G_i/G_o protein; K^+ = potassium; Na^+ = sodium; TH = tyrosine hydroxylase; cAMP = cyclic adenosine 3′,5′-monophosphate; CREB = cAMP response element binding.

zation caused by morphine (Carlezon et al. 1997), perhaps due to enhanced Ca^{2+} permeability of channels composed of GluR1 subunits and located on VTA dopamine neurons. Thus, opioids might interact with mesolimbic dopamine neurons to produce reinforcement, especially given that the reinforcing properties of morphine are eliminated in mice lacking the D_2-like receptor (Maldonado et al. 1997).

Persistent Neuroadaptation During Withdrawal

Most substances that cause dependence also produce withdrawal symptoms, which can be somatic, affective, or behavioral in nature. In fact, these symptom types may coexist at particular times during withdrawal due to the concurrent involvement of different brain systems. Somatic symptoms are most easily recognized, producing physical withdrawal in cases of opioid or alcohol dependence. Cocaine or amphetamine withdrawal produces dysphoric or depressive symptoms, especially following binge exposure, and leads to persistent changes in brain chemistry with profound functional consequences.

Opioid withdrawal is largely the result of hyperactivity of noradrenergic LC neurons due to increased cAMP signaling and excitatory stimulation of the LC. Chronic opioid exposure leads to compensatory changes in channels permitting normal cellular activity in the presence of sustained opioid inhibition, as described above (see also Figure 4–3, right). Following chronic opioid treatment, elimination of opioids or treatment with an opioid antagonist reduces opioid receptor stimulation. Enhanced LC neuronal activity then remains unopposed, and the resulting hyperexcitability of LC neurons precipitates withdrawal symptoms by stimulating sympathetic activity and inducing anxiety.

Although LC hyperactivity might explain some of the somatic and affective symptoms lasting for several days after opioid withdrawal, additional brain regions affected either by noradrenergic hyperactivity or by reduced opioid stimulation could account for other symptoms during withdrawal. For example, hyperactivity of the GABAergic interneurons that express μ receptors in the VTA could inhibit firing of mesolimbic dopamine neurons during opioid withdrawal (Diana et al. 1999), resulting in dysphoria, irritability, and restlessness that can last for weeks. Aversive and anxiogenic states during withdrawal also might be the result of activation of corticotropin-releasing factor (CRF)–containing neurons in the amygdala (Koob and Heinrichs 1999).

Psychostimulants produce withdrawal symptoms that differ from those of opioids but that nevertheless cause significant and severe impairment. Binge cocaine self-administration followed by drug withdrawal produces reductions in NAc dopamine and serotonin levels (Parsons et al. 1995), elevated thresholds for intracranial electrical self-stimulation (Markou and Koob 1991), and increased distress calls in rodent models (Mutschler and Miczek 1998). These animal model correlates are associated with symptoms experienced during the early "crash" phase of cocaine withdrawal in humans (Gawin 1991). Enhancement of the cAMP pathway and accumulation of chronic ΔFosB results in persistent dynorphin expression in the striatum that might serve to limit the activation of striatal neurons (Steiner and Gerfen 1998). These effects lead to a long-lasting depression of NAc metabolic activity and immediate-early gene expression lasting for weeks after cessation of cocaine self-administration in animals (Hammer et al. 1993; Onton and Hammer 2000) and humans (Volkow et al. 1992). Animals trained to self-administer cocaine also exhibit a profound reduction of the transcription factor *zif268* in the hippocampus and amygdala during withdrawal (Mutschler et al. 2000). Given that synaptic modifications required for neuronal plasticity and learning are thought to be stabilized by *zif268* (Hughes et al. 1999), relearning to avoid conditioned drug responses could be even more difficult to achieve during withdrawal. Thus, cocaine-dependent individuals might be "doomed" to relapse to conditioned drug-taking behavior unless the biochemical basis for this deficit can be corrected.

Augmented behavioral sensitization induced by repeated psychostimulant use can affect both the type and the magnitude of drug response during withdrawal. For example, chronic cocaine use may lead to transient paranoia upon subsequent reexposure in up to two-thirds of cocaine-dependent individuals (Satel et al. 1991). During withdrawal, behavioral sensitization is generally augmented for several weeks after cessation of cocaine self-administration in animals, suggesting that conditioned behavioral responses might recur after the initial crash phase of withdrawal. In fact, prior cocaine self-administration enhances the reinstatement of higher cocaine intake during withdrawal in animals (Deroche et al. 1999). Behavioral sensitization during cocaine withdrawal depends on increased NAc glutamate level as a result of enhanced activity of corticostriatal projections from limbic forebrain regions (Hammer and Cooke 1996; Pierce et al. 1996). Cocaine-dependent individuals viewing a videotape showing paraphernalia associated with cocaine use (cocaine-conditioned cues) experience drug craving and activation of the anterior cingulate and amygdalar regions that supply the NAc (Childress et al. 1999). Furthermore, cocaine-conditioned cues increase NAc and amygdalar dopamine levels, which may be sufficient to stimulate reinstatement of self-administration (Weiss et al. 2000). The most intense stimuli for reinstatement of drug-seeking behavior are reexposure to the drug and exposure to stress (Stewart 2000). Repeated exposure to an intense social stressor produces persistent upregulation of μ receptor mRNA expression in VTA interneurons (Nikulina et al. 1999), thereby disinhibiting the mesolimbic dopamine pathway upon subsequent exposure to the drug. Therefore, such stress-induced cross-sensitization could enhance subjects' vulnerability for initiating drug self-administration in the future, because drug-naïve individuals would be "presensitized" by prior stress exposure.

Withdrawal from other substances seems to affect biochemical substrates similar to those involved in opioid and cocaine withdrawal, although regional specificity might exist. Abrupt cessation of chronic alcohol administration profoundly reduces NAc dopamine (Diana et al. 1993), which is restored by subsequent reinstatement of alcohol self-administration (Weiss et al. 1996). Chronic alcohol exposure also upregulates the cAMP pathway, desensitizes $GABA_A$ receptors, and increases NMDA receptor expression. Alcohol appears to release endogenous opioids, as naltrexone reduces alcohol reinforcement. Naloxone can precipitate withdrawal symptoms following chronic cannabinoid treatment (Navarro et al. 1998), which selectively upregulates the cAMP pathway in the cerebellum, leading to impairment of motor coordination (Tzavara et al. 2000). Opioid antagonists also block the effects of nicotine and increase withdrawal symptoms in nicotine-dependent individuals.

For nicotine, the mechanism of adaptation differs but the ultimate effect is similar. Acute nicotine exposure stimulates nicotinic receptors, opening a ligand-gated cation channel to transiently increase sodium and potassium permeability. This stimulates neuronal activity in various brain regions, including the NAc and amygdala (Stein et al. 1998). Continued nicotine exposure produces desensitization and eventual upregulation of nicotine receptors. Gradual reduction of plasma nicotine level during short-term withdrawal permits receptor resensitization and hyperexcitability of cholinergic systems, producing anxiety, discomfort, and nicotine craving that is relieved by the next nicotine dose (cigarette). The greatest impact on both reduction of such withdrawal symptoms and reinforcement may come from the first cigarette of the day after a period of abstinence during sleep, when receptor resensitization and hyperexcitability is maximal. Nicotine withdrawal also reduces extracellular dopamine levels in both the NAc and the amygdala (Panagis et al. 2000), an effect that might underlie craving and other symptoms (e.g., anxiety, autonomic signs).

Functional Circuitry of Addiction

It is tempting to equate reinforcement with pleasure or hedonia, concluding that both are the result of mesolimbic dopamine enhancement. However, experimental animals in which the NAc is completely depleted of dopamine are still able to distinguish preferred foods, even though they become aphagic (Berridge and Robinson 1998). These dopamine-deficient animals know what they like, but apparently no longer desire food. Similarly, pimozide reduces amphetamine-induced *craving* in human subjects, whereas *euphoria* is unaffected (Brauer and

De Wit 1997). This has led to the conclusion that dopamine conveys the motivational value or "incentive salience" of a stimulus rather than encoding hedonia. This interpretation implies that dopaminergic stimulation of the NAc might induce craving (i.e., wanting or seeking). In fact, cocaine-induced activation of the NAc assessed by using functional magnetic resonance imaging (fMRI) in cocaine-dependent subjects is correlated with craving rather than with subjective "rush" or euphoria (Breiter et al. 1997). Dopamine, therefore, can be viewed as signaling motivation to the forebrain reward circuit. Dopamine might not be the only trigger for drug-related behaviors, however, given that conditioned responses can be elicited even in the presence of dopamine blockade. Activation of NAc AMPA or dopamine receptors produces reinstatement of cocaine self-administration during withdrawal in experimental animals, but cocaine- or AMPA-induced reinstatement is unaffected by fluphenazine, a dopamine receptor antagonist (Cornish and Kalivas 2000). Thus, stimulation of NAc AMPA receptors by glutamate derived from various sources is necessary and sufficient to elicit responding in an individual conditioned to self-administer cocaine. Dopamine might serve to motivate drug responding upon initial exposure, and then exacerbate subsequent conditioned responding.

Normally, conditioned drug cues stimulate the amygdala and prefrontal limbic cortical regions (Childress et al. 1999), both of which provide glutamatergic input to the NAc. Amygdalar lesions prevent reinstatement of self-administration caused by drug-related stimuli and block the ability to associate stimuli with reinforcement value (Malkova et al. 1997; Meil and See 1997). The amygdala also responds to negative affect or conditioned aversive stimuli, so amygdalar input could convey various dimensions of drug-related emotional content to the NAc, especially during withdrawal. The orbital and medial prefrontal cortical areas, which also receive mesocortical dopamine input, process motivational cues to determine goal-directed behavioral outcomes related to abused substances as well as food and probably other addictive stimuli (Ongur and Price 2000). The hippocampus and ventral subiculum provide the contextual background on which conditioned reinforcement depends (Everitt et al. 1999). Cortical input from these various sources converges on individual NAc neurons (Wright and Groenewegen 1995), and hippocampal contributions may regulate the effect of prefrontal input by inducing a depolarized state in selected NAc neurons (O'Donnell and Grace 1995). The NAc, then, serves to integrate the emotional nature and the intended direction with the contextual condition (each conveyed by glutamatergic input), which can then be amplified by appropriate motivation (modulated by dopamine) to produce *action* via specific NAc afferent pathways (Figure 4–4).

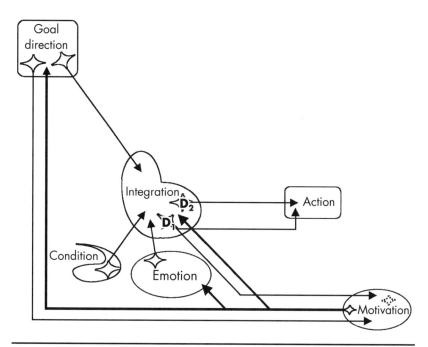

Figure 4–4. *Functional circuitry of addiction. This illustration of the neural circuits underlying reinforcement shows the functional impact of various efferent and afferent connections of the nucleus accumbens, which integrates incoming data to produce various outcomes (e.g., behavioral, emotional, cognitive). Mesolimbic dopamine conveys the motivational or incentive value of a stimulus, but conditioned reinforcement can be elicited even in the absence of dopamine. Glutamate input from cortical regions probably becomes increasingly important in stimulating conditioned responses and relapse during withdrawal. Cortical regions add various dimensions of context to integrated responses. Amygdalar input conveys emotional associations, and the hippocampus serves as a comparator of the relevant contextual condition and governs the goal direction contributed by input from prefrontal regions.*

Although the NAc might be the integrative center of the forebrain addiction circuit, it represents only one stop in a complex cortico-striato-pallido-thalamo-cortical loop (see Figure 4–1). This reverberatory circuit can be considered to be the neuroadaptive core of dependence. Within this circuit, abundant opportunities exist for neural plasticity through which new patterns of motivated behavior (e.g., conditioned drug seeking, compulsive substance use) or response (e.g., craving) are generated. Normally, environmental exposure alters brain substrates so as to better respond to related experiences. In the case of exogenous substances that powerfully stimulate endogenous reward circuits, a series of compensatory responses might inadvertently produce dysphoria, anxiety, or other undesirable symptoms, causing the individual to seek and sustain substance abuse.

Some individuals exhibit an intrinsic vulnerability to the use or response to abused substances. Animals that prefer alcohol are more sensitive to the effects of repeated cocaine or morphine administration, and strains of animals that exhibit intrinsic induction of the cAMP pathway in the NAc (e.g., Lewis rats) more readily acquire cocaine self-administration (Honkanen et al. 1999; Kosten et al. 1997). Furthermore, the magnitude of an individual's response to alcohol, as well as certain personality characteristics with heretofore unknown genetic and biological bases, may determine his or her vulnerability to alcohol or drug dependence (Cloninger 1994; Schuckit 1998). Thus, specific biological factors determine the probability that addiction will develop following first exposure to a substance, including 1) the intrinsic state of the biological substrate affected by the substance, 2) the magnitude of response within reward circuits, and 3) the degree of neural adaptations occurring as a consequence of initial exposure. In contrast to earlier dogma, the distinct pathophysiology of addiction described here suggests that subsequent drug-seeking and self-administration behavior will be decreasingly dependent on choice and increasingly driven by adaptive biological changes in reward circuits. The onset of a progressive disease process ultimately produces compulsive behaviors that underlie dependence. However, the biological trigger for uncontrollable substance use, invoking behavioral and autonomic dysregulation (Tornatzky and Miczek 2000) and presumably differentiating abuse from dependence, remains unresolved.

Psychopharmacology

The mechanisms of acute action of abused substances vary considerably, with different substances affecting different receptors, transporters, and/or signaling substrates. The treatment of addiction, however, ultimately must involve more than just correction of this initial mechanism. Virtually all abused substances affect various elements of the functional circuitry of addiction (see Figure 4–4), producing intracellular neuroadaptive changes that often result in tolerance to the desired subjective effects. At the same time, additional elements of this circuitry give rise to sensitization, conditioned responses, and undesirable mood changes, while adaptations in other brain regions can produce autonomic and somatic symptoms. These multiple regional and neurochemical effects of repeated exposure to substances of abuse suggest that no simple solution to addiction will be forthcoming. Instead, continuing research is likely to identify unique molecular targets for distinct stages of abuse, dependence, and withdrawal that exhibit common adaptations across different abused substances.

Most current therapeutic interventions apply recent knowledge of the brain substrates altered by chronic exposure. In some cases, symptomatic treatment related to specific drug effects can be useful. For example, sympathetic hyperactivity and anxiety symptoms can be attenuated by stimulation of α_2-adrenergic autoreceptors using clonidine, presumably by reducing LC neuronal firing and norepinephrine release. The partial opioid agonist buprenorphine can be used to provide limited opioid replacement during withdrawal while blocking the effect of higher exogenous opioid levels. Naltrexone, a full opioid antagonist, also reduces alcohol craving in alcohol dependence and withdrawal, presumably by blocking endogenous opioids.

Recent data suggest that other approaches may be used to effectively treat addiction to various substances of abuse, depending on the specific stage of addiction. For example, chronic use of alcohol, cocaine, opioids, and nicotine is known to reduce NAc dopamine during early withdrawal, so the selective dopamine and norepinephrine reuptake inhibitor bupropion might relieve craving or depressed mood during this period. It is possible that continued bupropion treatment might facilitate readjustment of an altered "set point" for NAc function. Alternatively, bupropion might act during the recovery stage to promote reinstatement of self-administration, given that it is known to be reinforcing and to substitute for psychostimulants in drug discrimination trials. Dopamine function also can be enhanced during early withdrawal by using the monoamine oxidase B inhibitor selegiline. Alcohol and opioid withdrawal enhance NAc glutamate release and NMDA receptor sensitivity, which has led to the use of acamprosate, a taurine derivative, to modulate glutamatergic hyperactivity during withdrawal. Another possible means of inhibiting striatal glutamatergic activity is through administration of direct or indirect adenosine receptor agonists, which reduce opioid withdrawal symptoms (Kaplan and Coyle 1998; Kaplan and Sears 1996). Such attempts to depress glutamatergic activity during early withdrawal must be weighed against the apparent need for AMPA receptor activation during recovery in the NAc. GluR1 subunit expression is induced in the NAc during successful extinction from cocaine self-administration, and experimental induction of NAc GluR1 expression reduces cocaine-seeking behavior during extinction (Schmidt et al. 1999). Therefore, glutamate action at NAc AMPA receptors might be essential for neural plasticity and relearning of appropriate non-drug-responding behavior during recovery from addiction.

Thus, the stage of exposure, whether abuse, dependence, early withdrawal, recovery, or relapse, might be a particularly important determinant of treatment approach. Common adaptations occurring within specific reward regions may provide viable substrates for pharmacotherapy when used during the correct stage of addiction. Furthermore, the efficacy of pharmacotherapy during the recovery stage might be enhanced by concurrent behavioral therapy to facilitate the development of therapeutic neuroplasticity in reward circuits. Research on the circuitry and signaling of addiction is just beginning to yield rewards.

References

American Psychiatric Association: Diagnostic and Statistical Manual of Mental Disorders, 4th Edition, Text Revision. Washington, DC, American Psychiatric Association, 2000

Beitner-Johnson D, Guitart X, Nestler EJ: Dopaminergic brain reward regions of Lewis and Fischer rats display different levels of tyrosine hydroxylase and other morphine- and cocaine-regulated phosphoproteins. Brain Res 561: 147–150, 1991

Berridge KC, Robinson TE: What is the role of dopamine in reward: hedonic impact, reward learning, or incentive salience? Brain Res Brain Res Rev 28: 309–369, 1998

Brauer LH, De Wit H: High dose pimozide does not block amphetamine-induced euphoria in normal volunteers. Pharmacol Biochem Behav 56:265–272, 1997

Breiter HC, Gollub RL, Weisskoff RM, et al: Acute effects of cocaine on human brain activity and emotion. Neuron 19:591–611, 1997

Calabresi P, Centonze D, Gubellini P, et al: Synaptic transmission in the striatum: from plasticity to neurodegeneration. Prog Neurobiol 61:231–265, 2000

Carlezon WA, Boundy VA, Haile CN, et al: Sensitization to morphine induced by viral-mediated gene transfer. Science 277:812–814, 1997

Carlezon WA, Thome J, Olson VG, et al: Regulation of cocaine reward by CREB. Science 282:2272–2275, 1998

Cepeda C, Levine MS: Dopamine and N-methyl-D-aspartate receptor interactions in the neostriatum. Dev Neurosci 20:1–18, 1998

Chergui K, Nomikos GG, Math JM, et al: Burst stimulation of the medial forebrain bundle selectively increases Fos-like immunoreactivity in the limbic forebrain of the rat. Neuroscience 72:141–156, 1996

Childress AR, Mozley PD, McElgin W, et al: Limbic activation during cue-induced cocaine craving. Am J Psychiatry 156:11–18, 1999

Churchill L, Swanson CJ, Urbina M, et al: Repeated cocaine alters glutamate receptor subunit levels in the nucleus accumbens and ventral tegmental area of rats that develop behavioral sensitization. J Neurochem 72:2397–2403, 1999

Cloninger CR: Temperament and personality. Curr Opin Neurobiol 4:266–273, 1994

Cornish JL, Kalivas PW: Glutamate transmission in the nucleus accumbens mediates relapse in cocaine addiction. J Neurosci 20:RC89, 2000 [online article—Rapid Communication (RC)—available at http://www.jneurosci.org/cgi/content/full/20/15/RC89]

Cornish JL, Duffy P, Kalivas PW: A role for nucleus accumbens glutamate transmission in the relapse to cocaine-seeking behavior. Neuroscience 93:1359–1367, 1999

Deroche V, Le Moal M, Piazza PV: Cocaine self-administration increases the incentive motivational properties of the drug in rats. Eur J Neurosci 11:2731–2736, 1999

Di Chiara G: A motivational learning hypothesis of the role of mesolimbic dopamine in compulsive drug use. J Psychopharmacol 12:54–67, 1998

Diana M, Pistis M, Carboni S, et al: Profound decrement of mesolimbic dopaminergic neuronal activity during ethanol withdrawal syndrome in rats: electrophysiological and biochemical evidence. Proc Natl Acad Sci U S A 90:7966–7969, 1993

Diana M, Muntoni AL, Pistis M, et al: Lasting reduction in mesolimbic dopamine neuronal activity after morphine withdrawal. Eur J Neurosci 11:1037–1041, 1999

Dirckx JH (ed): Stedman's Concise Medical Dictionary for the Health Professions, 3rd Edition. Baltimore, MD, Williams & Wilkins, 1997

Everitt BJ, Parkinson JA, Olmstead MC, et al: Associative processes in addiction and reward: the role of amygdala-ventral striatal subsystems. Ann N Y Acad Sci 877:412–438, 1999

Ferre S, Popoli P, Tinner-Staines B, et al: Adenosine A_1 receptor–dopamine D_1 receptor interaction in the rat limbic system: modulation of dopamine D_1 receptor antagonist binding sites. Neurosci Lett 208:109–112, 1996

Fiorino DF, Coury A, Fibiger HC, et al: Electrical stimulation of reward sites in the ventral tegmental area increases dopamine transmission in the nucleus accumbens of the rat. Behav Brain Res 55:131–141, 1993

Fitzgerald LW, Ortiz J, Hamedani AG, et al: Drugs of abuse and stress increase the expression of GluR1 and NMDAR1 glutamate receptor subunits in the rat ventral tegmental area: common adaptations among cross-sensitizing agents. J Neurosci 16:274–282, 1996

Gallistel CR, Karras D: Pimozide and amphetamine have opposing effects on the reward summation function. Pharmacol Biochem Behav 20:73–77, 1984

Gawin FH: Cocaine addiction: psychology and neurophysiology. Science 251: 1580–1586, 1991

Gerfen CR, Keefe KA, Gauda EB: D_1 and D_2 dopamine receptor function in the striatum: coactivation of D_1- and D_2-dopamine receptors on separate populations of neurons results in potentiated immediate early gene response in D_1-containing neurons. J Neurosci 15:8167–8176, 1995

Hammer RP, Cooke ES: Sensitization of neuronal response to cocaine challenge during withdrawal following chronic treatment. Neuroreport 7:2041–2045, 1996

Hammer RP, Pires WS, Markou A, et al: Withdrawal following cocaine self-administration decreases regional cerebral metabolic rate in critical brain reward regions. Synapse 14:73–80, 1993

Hernández-Lopez S, Bargas J, Surmeier DJ, et al: D_1 receptor activation enhances evoked discharge in neostriatal medium spiny neurons by modulating an L-type Ca^{2+} conductance. J Neurosci 17:3334–3342, 1997

Honkanen A, Mikkola J, Korpi ER, et al: Enhanced morphine- and cocaine-induced behavioral sensitization in alcohol-preferring AA rats. Psychopharmacology (Berl) 142:244–252, 1999

Hughes PE, Alexi T, Walton M, et al: Activity and injury-dependent expression of inducible transcription factors, growth factors and apoptosis-related genes within the central nervous system. Prog Neurobiol 57:421–450, 1999

Hyman SE, Cole RL, Konradi C, et al: Dopamine regulation of transcription factor-target interactions in rat striatum. Chemical Senses 20:257–260, 1995

Jongen-Relo AL, Groenewegen HJ, Voorn P: Evidence for a multi-compartmental histochemical organization of the nucleus accumbens in the rat. J Comp Neurol 337:267–276, 1993

Kaplan GB, Coyle TS: Adenosine kinase inhibitors attenuate opiate withdrawal via adenosine receptor activation. Eur J Pharmacol 362:1–8, 1998

Kaplan GB, Sears MT: Adenosine receptor agonists attenuate and adenosine receptor antagonists exacerbate opiate withdrawal signs. Psychopharmacology (Berl) 123:64–70, 1996

Kelz MB, Chen J, Carlezon WA, et al: Expression of the transcription factor deltaFosB in the brain controls sensitivity to cocaine. Nature 401:272–276, 1999

Konradi C, Heckers S: Haloperidol-induced Fos expression in striatum is dependent upon transcription factor cyclic AMP response element binding protein. Neuroscience 65:1051–1061, 1995

Koob GF: The role of the striatopallidal and extended amygdala systems in drug addiction. Ann N Y Acad Sci 877: 445–460, 1999

Koob GF, Heinrichs SC: A role for corticotropin releasing factor and urocortin in behavioral responses to stressors. Brain Res 848:141–152, 1999

Kosten TA, Miserendino MJ, Haile CN, et al: Acquisition and maintenance of intravenous cocaine self-administration in Lewis and Fischer inbred rat strains. Brain Res 778:418–429, 1997

Lane-Ladd SB, Pineda J, Boundy VA, et al: CREB (cAMP response element-binding protein) in the locus coeruleus: biochemical, physiological, and behavioral evidence for a role in opiate dependence. J Neurosci 17:7890–7901, 1997

Le Moine C, Bloch B: D_1 and D_2 dopamine receptor gene expression in the rat striatum: sensitive cRNA probes demonstrate prominent segregation of D_1 and D_2 mRNAs in distinct neuronal populations of the dorsal and ventral striatum. J Comp Neurol 355:418–426, 1995

Ledent C, Valverde O, Cossu G, et al: Unresponsiveness to cannabinoids and reduced addictive effects of opiates in CB1 receptor knockout mice. Science 283:401–404, 1999

Leshner AI: Addiction is a brain disease, and it matters. Science 278:45–47, 1997

Maldonado R, Saiardi A, Valverde O, et al: Absence of opiate rewarding effects in mice lacking dopamine D_2 receptors. Nature 388:586–589, 1997

Malkova L, Gaffan D, Murray EA: Excitotoxic lesions of the amygdala fail to produce impairment in visual learning for auditory secondary reinforcement but interfere with reinforcer devaluation effects in rhesus monkeys. J Neurosci 17:6011–6020, 1997

Markou A, Koob GF: Postcocaine anhedonia. An animal model of cocaine withdrawal. Neuropsychopharmacology 4:17–26, 1991

Matthes HW, Maldonado R, Simonin F, et al: Loss of morphine-induced analgesia, reward effect and withdrawal symptoms in mice lacking the mu-opioid-receptor gene. Nature 383:819–823, 1996

Meil WM, See RE: Lesions of the basolateral amygdala abolish the ability of drug associated cues to reinstate responding during withdrawal from self-administered cocaine. Behav Brain Res 87:139–148, 1997

Mendelson JH, Sholar M, Mello NK, et al: Cocaine tolerance: behavioral, cardiovascular, and neuroendocrine function in men. Neuropsychopharmacology 18:263–271, 1998

Mutschler NH, Miczek KA: Withdrawal from i.v. cocaine "binges" in rats: ultrasonic distress calls and startle. Psychopharmacology (Berl) 135:161–168, 1998

Mutschler NH, Miczek KA, Hammer RP Jr: Reduction of *zif268* messenger RNA expression during prolonged withdrawal following "binge" cocaine self-administration in rats. Neuroscience 100:531–538, 2000

Navarro M, Chowen J, Carrera MRA, et al: CB1 cannabinoid receptor antagonist-induced opiate withdrawal in morphine-dependent rats. Neuroreport 9:3397–3402, 1998

Nestler EJ, Aghajanian GK: Molecular and cellular basis of addiction. Science 278:58–63, 1997

Nestler EJ, Terwilliger RZ, Walker JR, et al: Chronic cocaine treatment decreases levels of the G protein subunits G_i and G_o in discrete regions of rat brain. J Neurochem 55:1079–1082, 1990

Nestler EJ, Alreja M, Aghajanian GK: Molecular control of locus coeruleus neurotransmission. Biol Psychiatry 46:1131–1139, 1999a

Nestler EJ, Kelz MB, Chen J: ΔFosB: a molecular mediator of long-term neural and behavioral plasticity. Brain Res 835:10–17, 1999b

Nikulina EM, Hammer RP, Miczek KA, et al: Social defeat stress increases expression of μ-opioid receptor-encoding mRNA in the rat ventral tegmental area. Neuroreport 10:3015–3019, 1999

O'Donnell P, Grace AA: Synaptic interactions among excitatory afferents to nucleus accumbens neurons: hippocampal gating of prefrontal cortical input. J Neurosci 15:3622–3639, 1995

Ongur D, Price JL: The organization of networks within the orbital and medial prefrontal cortex of rats, monkeys and humans. Cereb Cortex 10:206–219, 2000

Onton J, Hammer RP: Behavioral sensitization is associated with reduced *zif268* mRNA expression in the nucleus accumbens during withdrawal following cocaine self-administration. Society for Neuroscience Abstracts 26:526, 2000

Ortiz J, Fitzgerald LW, Charlton M, et al: Biochemical actions of chronic ethanol exposure in the mesolimbic dopamine system. Synapse 21:289–298, 1995

Panagis G, Hildebrand BE, Svensson TH, et al: Selective c-fos induction and decreased dopamine release in the central nucleus of amygdala in rats displaying a mecamylamine-precipitated nicotine withdrawal syndrome. Synapse 35:15–25, 2000

Parsons LH, Koob GF, Weiss F: Serotonin dysfunction in the nucleus accumbens of rats during withdrawal after unlimited access to intravenous cocaine. J Pharmacol Exp Ther 274:1182–1191, 1995

Pierce RC, Bell K, Duffy P, et al: Repeated cocaine augments excitatory amino acid transmission in the nucleus accumbens only in rats having developed behavioral sensitization. J Neurosci 16:1550–1560, 1996

Pitcher JA, Freedman NJ, Lefkowitz RJ: G protein–coupled receptor kinases. Annu Rev Biochem 67:653–692, 1998

Rahman Z, Gold SJ, Potenza MN, et al: Cloning and characterization of RGS9-2: a striatal-enriched alternatively spliced product of the RGS9 gene. J Neurosci 19:2016–2026, 1999

Ritz MC, Lamb RJ, Goldberg SR, et al: Cocaine receptors on dopamine transporters are related to self-administration of cocaine. Science 237:1219–1223, 1987

Robertson GS, Jian M: D$_1$ and D$_2$ dopamine receptors differentially increase Fos-like immunoreactivity in accumbal projections to the ventral pallidum and midbrain. Neuroscience 64:1019–1034, 1995

Satel SL, Southwick SM, Gawin FH: Clinical features of cocaine-induced paranoia. Am J Psychiatry 148:495–498, 1991

Schmidt EF, Karanian DA, Schad CA, et al: Viral vector–mediated up-regulation of GluR1 AMPA/kainate receptor subunits in the nucleus accumbens reduces cocaine-seeking behavior during extinction. Society for Neuroscience Abstracts 25:813, 1999

Schuckit MA: Biological, psychological and environmental predictors of the alcoholism risk: a longitudinal study. J Stud Alcohol 59:485–494, 1998

Self DW, Terwilliger RZ, Nestler EJ, et al: Inactivation of G_i and G_o proteins in nucleus accumbens reduces both cocaine and heroin reinforcement. J Neurosci 14:6239–6247, 1994

Self DW, Genova LM, Hope BT, et al: Involvement of cAMP-dependent protein kinase in the nucleus accumbens in cocaine self-administration and relapse of cocaine-seeking behavior. J Neurosci 18:1848–1859, 1998

Stedman TL: Stedman's Medical Dictionary: A Vocabulary of Medicine and Its Allied Sciences, 23rd Edition. Baltimore, MD, Williams & Wilkins, 1977

Stein EA, Pankiewicz J, Harsch HH, et al: Nicotine-induced limbic cortical activation in the human brain: a functional MRI study. Am J Psychiatry 155: 1009–1015, 1998

Steiner H, Gerfen CR: Role of dynorphin and enkephalin in the regulation of striatal output pathways and behavior. Exp Brain Res 123:60–76, 1998

Stewart J: Pathways to relapse: the neurobiology of drug- and stress-induced relapse to drug-taking. J Psychiatry Neurosci 25:125–136, 2000

Terwilliger RZ, Beitner-Johnson D, Sevarino KA, et al: A general role for adaptations in G-proteins and the cyclic AMP system in mediating the chronic actions of morphine and cocaine on neuronal function. Brain Res 548:100–110, 1991

Thomas WL, Cooke ES, Hammer RP: Cocaine-induced sensitization of metabolic activity in extrapyramidal circuits involves prior D_1-like dopamine receptor stimulation. J Pharmacol Exp Ther 278:347–353, 1996

Tornatzky W, Miczek KA: Cocaine self-administration "binges": transition from behavioral and autonomic regulation toward homeostatic dysregulation in rats. Psychopharmacology (Berl) 148:289–298, 2000

Tzavara ET, Valjent E, Firmo C, et al: Cannabinoid withdrawal is dependent upon PKA activation in the cerebellum. Eur J Neurosci 12:1038–1046, 2000

Volkow ND, Hitzemann R, Wang G-J, et al: Long-term frontal brain metabolic changes in cocaine abusers. Synapse 11:184–190, 1992

Voorn P, Brady LS, Berendse HW, et al: Densitometrical analysis of opioid receptor ligand binding in the human striatum, I: distribution of μ opioid receptor defines shell and core of the ventral striatum. Neuroscience 75:777–792, 1996

Weiss F, Parsons LH, Schulteis G, et al: Ethanol self-administration restores withdrawal-associated deficiencies in accumbal dopamine and 5-hydroxytryptamine release in dependent rats. J Neurosci 16:3474–3485, 1996

Weiss F, Maldonado-Vlaar CS, Parsons LH, et al: Control of cocaine-seeking behavior by drug-associated stimuli in rats: effects on recovery of extinguished operant-responding and extracellular dopamine levels in amygdala and nucleus accumbens. Proc Natl Acad Sci U S A 97:4321–4326, 2000

Whistler JL, Chuang HH, Chu P, et al: Functional dissociation of µ opioid receptor signaling and endocytosis: implications for the biology of opiate tolerance and addiction. Neuron 23:737–746, 1999

Wright CI, Groenewegen HJ: Patterns of convergence and segregation in the medial nucleus accumbens of the rat: relationships of prefrontal cortical, midline thalamic, and basal amygdaloid afferents. J Comp Neurol 361:383–403, 1995

CHAPTER 5

Neural Circuitry and Signaling in Anxiety

Justine M. Kent, M.D.
Gregory M. Sullivan, M.D.
Scott L. Rauch, M.D.

O ver the past two decades, neurobiological research in the field of anxiety has provided a wealth of new information regarding neural pathways relevant to the behavioral and physiological expression of normal and pathological anxiety. Current neuroanatomic and neurochemical hypotheses of anxiety have been informed by preclinical research using animal models of fear, stress, and anxiety and by biological and pharmacological challenge studies in humans, which have identified behavioral, neuroendocrine, and autonomic response abnormalities in subjects with anxiety disorders. Neuroimaging techniques are currently being used to test neuroanatomic hypotheses derived from animal and clinical studies. These methods have resulted in a new view of the anxiety disorders, one based not only on their symptomatology and treatment response, but also on evolving models of their underlying pathophysiology. A comprehensive review of the neurobiology of each anxiety disorder is beyond the scope of this chapter. Therefore, we limit our discussion to current hypotheses regarding neurocircuitry and signaling pathways for those anxiety disorders that have been best studied from a neurobiological perspective: panic disorder, posttraumatic stress disorder, and obsessive-compulsive disorder.

Clinical Presentation

Symptom overlap in the anxiety disorders is extensive, and comorbidity with other anxiety disorders, depression, and substance abuse is more the rule than the exception. However, despite symptom commonality, each anxiety disorder is distinguished by a set of operationalized criteria specific to that disorder.

Panic attacks, the core clinical feature of panic disorder, are defined as the rapid onset of intense fear or discomfort in a crescendo pattern, accompanied by distressing somatic and/or cognitive symptoms. Somatic symptoms typically involve activation of the respiratory, cardiac, and gastrointestinal systems, whereas cognitive symptoms focus on specific fears, such as losing control, going crazy, or dying. Attacks are generally short-lived but cause tremendous distress and are often accompanied by an intense desire to flee the situation in which the attack occurs. Attacks may also be accompanied by symptoms of depersonalization or derealization.

Panic disorder is characterized by the occurrence of spontaneous panic attacks, resulting in persistent worry about having another attack and avoidance of situations in which an attack is felt likely or feared. Spontaneous panic attacks are often interspersed with situationally predisposed panic attacks involving crowds, subways, bridges, and the like. Phobic avoidance may generalize to situations unrelated to or only loosely connected to the original situation where panic occurred, resulting in *agoraphobia*. Agoraphobia is a severe form of phobic avoidance, occurring in approximately 30% of patients with panic disorder, that involves a more general anxiety about being in places or situations in which a panic attack may occur and in which help or an escape route may not be immediately available.

Posttraumatic stress disorder (PTSD) is characterized by a particular constellation of symptoms that develop in the aftermath of an emotionally traumatic event. By definition, the traumatic event has involved threat of death, injury, or bodily harm to oneself or others. The person's response to the traumatic event must be one of intense fear or helplessness. The resulting symptoms are divided into three categories: reexperiencing, persistent avoidance, and hyperarousal. *Reexperiencing* symptoms include recurrent, intrusive recollections, nightmares, and flashbacks (the vivid reliving of the traumatic event). *Persistent avoidance* symptoms include an effort to avoid trauma-related thoughts or feelings, along with avoidance of trauma-related activities, situations, or people. This may involve detachment from others, accompanied by psychological numbing, diminished interest in activities, and the sense of a foreshortened future. *Hyperarousal* symptoms include difficulty concentrating, hypervigilance, increased irritability, exaggerated startle, sleep disturbances, and difficulty modulating affect (particularly anger).

Obsessive-compulsive disorder (OCD) is characterized by the presence of intrusive thoughts or impulses (*obsessions*). The obsessions are typically accompanied by anxiety, which in turn prompts behaviors (*compulsions*) that are performed in a ritualized fashion in an effort to neutralize the obsessions and/or their attendant anxiety. Persons with OCD retain insight; they recognize that the obsessions are products of their own mind and that both obsessions and compulsions are excessive. Obsessions tend to fall into broad categories according to content: contamination, checking/ordering/counting, sexual impulses or imagery, and aggressive or harmful impulses, among others. Obsessions and compulsions cause marked distress and consume significant amounts of time, interfering with social and occupational functioning.

Neural Circuitry

Models of Fear and Anxiety

Fear accompanied by escape or avoidant behavior is an emotional/behavioral state that is present across animal species. Conditioned fear, in terms of physiological and behavioral response, is probably our best current model for anxiety disorders, despite its limitations. For instance, although most animal models of anxiety states involve conditioning, it is not clear that any anxiety disorder (except for PTSD) involves prior exposure to any aversive stimulus. Nevertheless, there are many features of conditioned fear in animals that make the analogy with anxiety disorders compelling. Thus, the neuroanatomy of conditioned fear in rodents has been used as a starting point for investigating the neurocircuitry of pathological fear in humans.

The critical pathways implicated in preclinical models of conditioned fear (Davis 1992; LeDoux et al. 1988) are shown in Figure 5–1. Sensory inputs from visual, auditory, olfactory, nociceptive, and visceral pathways run through the anterior thalamus to the lateral nucleus of the amygdala, which communicates with the central nucleus of the amygdala (CNA) (LeDoux et al. 1990). The CNA acts as the central point for the output of information, coordinating the autonomic and behavioral response to fear (Davis 1992; LeDoux et al. 1990). CNA efferents have many targets: the parabrachial nucleus, producing an increase in respiratory rate (Takeuchi et al. 1982); the lateral hypothalamus, activating the sympathetic nervous system and causing autonomic arousal and sympathetic discharge (Price and Amaral 1981); the locus coeruleus, resulting in an increase in norepinephrine release, which contributes to an increase in blood pressure and heart rate and the behavioral fear response (Cedarbaum and Aghajanian 1978); and the paraventricular nucleus of the hypothalamus, causing activation of

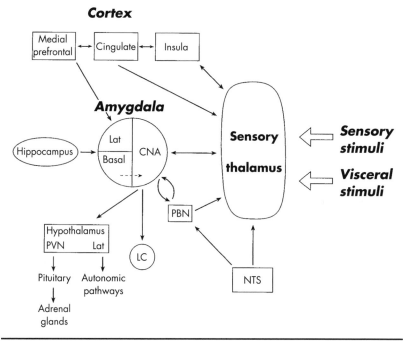

Figure 5–1. *Important pathways in fear conditioning. Sensory inputs run through the anterior thalamus to the lateral nucleus of the amygdala, which then communicates with the central nucleus of the amygdala (CNA). The CNA integrates the outputs and coordinates the autonomic and behavioral responses of fear. CNA efferents have many targets: to the parabrachial nucleus (PBN), producing an increase in respiratory rate; to the lateral hypothalamus, activating the sympathetic nervous system; to the locus coeruleus (LC), resulting in an increase in blood pressure and heart rate and the behavioral fear response; and to the paraventricular nucleus of the hypothalamus (PVN), causing activation of the hypothalamic-pituitary-adrenal (HPA) axis and resulting in an increase in adrenocorticoids. Lat = lateral; NTS = nucleus of the solitary tract.*

the hypothalamic-pituitary-adrenal (HPA) axis, which results in an increase in the release of adrenocorticoids (Dunn and Whitener 1986). A projection from the CNA to the periaqueductal gray (PAG) region is responsible for additional behavioral responses, including defensive behaviors and freezing, as well as pain modulation (De Oca et al. 1998).

The hippocampus is also thought to play a role in conditioned fear; the hippocampus processes information related to the context in which the fear cue is presented (Kim and Fanselow 1992). Preclinical studies suggest that the processes of cue and contextual fear conditioning are mediated by different amygdalar pathways. Sensory information regarding the conditioned stimulus (cue) is relayed through the thalamus and then converges with information about the unconditioned stimulus on the lateral nucleus of the amygdala before being transferred to the CNA. In contrast, contextual information appears to require the hippocampus to first create a representation of the environment using information received from the entorhinal cortex and subiculum (LeDoux et al. 1990). This information regarding context is relayed through the basal/accessory basal nuclei of the amygdala and then to the CNA. Thus, lesions of the lateral nucleus have been shown to block cue fear conditioning (LeDoux et al. 1990), whereas lesions of the basal/accessory nuclei attenuate contextual fear conditioning but have no effect on cue fear conditioning (Majidishad et al. 1996). One could imagine that deficits in hippocampal memory processing, or dysfunction in other elements of this system, would result in poor contextual stimulus discrimination, with resultant overgeneralization of fear responding, as seen in anxiety disorders.

There are important reciprocal connections between the amygdala and the sensory thalamus, the prefrontal cortex, and the insula and primary somatosensory cortex (de Olmos 1990). These connections allow the amygdala two major modes of responding: a rapid mode, based on direct input from the sensory thalamus, and a slower mode, based on pathways from the thalamus to the cortex to the amygdala (referred to by LeDoux [1996] as the "low road" and "high road," respectively). If the rapid mode, which is necessary for prompt response to immediate danger, is activated indiscriminately (i.e., without regard for the degree of danger), appropriate cortical assessment cannot take place and inappropriate threat responsiveness occurs. Such indiscriminate activation might result from insufficient constraint on the rapid thalamo-amygdalar path or deficits in the thalamo-cortico-amygdalar pathway. Although much remains to be learned regarding the amygdala's role in anxiety, pathological anxiety may reflect a deficit in the coordination of "top-down" (slower/thalamo-cortico-amygdalar) and/or "bottom-up" (rapid/thalamo-amygdalar) sensory information processing, leading to heightened amygdalar activity with resultant behavioral, autonomic, and neuroendocrine activation.

Clinical studies also point to the importance of the amygdala in human emotional perception and expression of fear. Lesions of the amygdala result in impaired recognition of fearful facial expressions (Adolphs et al. 1994) and impaired fear conditioning (Bechara et al. 1995), whereas electrical stimulation of the amygdala precipitates fearful, panic-like emotional responses (Halgren et al. 1978). Neuroimaging methods have recently enabled investigators to explore the neural substrates of these phenomena in humans, providing information regarding comparative functional anatomy. Several groups have demonstrated increased regional cerebral blood flow (rCBF) in the amygdala of healthy subjects in response to the presentation of fearful facial expressions (Whalen et al. 1998). Aversive classical (fear) conditioning paradigms in healthy human subjects produce activation in several subcortical structures implicated in the fear pathway, including the thalamus, hypothalamus, and PAG, as well as the somatosensory, cingulate, and association cortex (LaBar et al. 1998). One study demonstrated activation of the amygdala and periamygdaloid cortex during conditioned fear acquisition and extinction (LaBar et al. 1998).

Pharmacological challenge paradigms have also been used to explore the mediating anatomy of induced fear states. During procaine-induced complex emotional states, which include fear or anxiety as one component, anterior paralimbic and amygdala activation has been observed in healthy subjects (Ketter et al. 1996). The more selective panicogen cholecystokinin-4 (CCK-4) has also been used in functional imaging studies to elicit anxiety in healthy populations. In fact, two studies have demonstrated increased rCBF in the claustrum-insular-amygdalar region and the anterior cingulate during CCK-4 versus control infusions (Javanmard et al. 1999). One of these studies examined the change in rCBF as a function of time in healthy volunteers during CCK-induced panic (Javanmard et al. 1999). Results suggest that rCBF reduction in the medial frontal cortex occurred throughout, whereas specific early effects involved increases in rCBF in the hypothalamic region, and specific peak effects involved increases in the claustrum-insular region. These data may be viewed as consistent with activation of the brain stem–hypothalamic region via the thalamo-amygdalar circuit (fast circuit) followed by thalamo-cortical activation (slow circuit).

Neural Circuitry of Panic Disorder

Positron-emission tomography (PET) studies of patients with panic disorder in the absence of panic attack have suggested a possible abnormality in limbic (particularly hippocampal and parahippocampal) regions (Reiman et al. 1984). Despite the inherent challenges in attempting to elicit and image an acute, transient event such as a panic attack, several investigators have attempted challenge studies in concert with imaging in panic disorder. Two single photon emission computed tomography (SPECT) studies using symptom provocation paradigms indicated that patients with panic disorder may exhibit a decrease in widespread cortical (mainly frontal) cerebral blood flow (CBF) during panic episodes (Stewart et al. 1988). One PET study (Reiman et al. 1989) found rCBF increases in insular cortex and the claustrum/lateral putamen during lactate infusions. These limited functional neuroimaging data provide a picture of limbic/paralimbic activation together with frontal deactivation that may represent an exaggerated version of the profile seen in healthy subjects during various anxious states.

In regard to the general fear neurocircuitry described above, potential deficits in frontal cortical processing could lead to the misinterpretation of sensory information (bodily cues) known to be a hallmark of panic disorder, resulting in inappropriate activation of the fear network via misguided excitatory input to the amygdala. Thus, although the role of the amygdala in panic has yet to be elucidated, it seems likely that there is a deficit in the coordination and processing of top-down (cortical) and/or bottom-up (brain stem) sensory information, activating what may be a hyperresponsive amygdala.

Neural Circuitry of Posttraumatic Stress Disorder

In contrast to panic disorder, the heightened threat responsiveness in PTSD is to external cues and situations rather than to the internal cues (manifesting as feared bodily sensations) typical of panic disorder. Thus, in several respects, the development of PTSD is more easily likened to fear conditioning than the development of panic disorder. By definition, PTSD involves exposure to extreme threat that subsequently becomes associated with a constellation of situational factors. The individual then responds to reminders of those situational factors as if they are predictors of recurring threat. The main pathological aspects of PTSD—*overgeneralization of fear responding* to a wide range of reminders and *failure of extinction of the response*—have guided neurocircuitry models of PTSD pathophysiology. Such contemporary models of PTSD have focused on the relationships between the amygdala, hippocampus, and medial prefrontal cortex, the same triad of structures implicated in fear conditioning. More specifically, current theories have suggested some combination of hyperresponsivity of the amygdala to threat-related stimuli, and/or insufficient modulating influences from the hippocampus and/or medial prefrontal cortex. Hyperresponsivity within the amygdala might correspond to a liability for developing PTSD (i.e., extreme aptitude for fear conditioning) or it might represent a state marker corresponding to exaggerated threat responsiveness, hypervigilance, and enhanced startle. Likewise, inadequate hippocampal function might predispose to the development of PTSD or mediate overgeneralization of the threat response to innocuous contexts. Finally, inadequate top-down governance of the amygdala by the medial prefrontal cortex could represent the neural substrate for the failure to extinguish.

Neuroimaging studies have provided compelling data with regard to neurocircuitry models of PTSD. First, clinical morphometric magnetic resonance imaging (MRI) studies support hippocampal volume reduction in PTSD (Bremner et al. 1995). Furthermore, magnetic resonance spectroscopy (MRS) has been used to measure relative concentrations of N-acetyl aspartate (NAA) within the brain as a putative marker of neuron viability. Schuff and colleagues (1997) found nonsignificantly smaller (–6%) right hippocampal volumes in the PTSD group versus the control group on morphometric MRI and an 18% reduction in right hippocampal NAA concentrations with MRS. Although this study must be viewed as preliminary, it suggests that the smaller hippocampal volumes observed in PTSD patients may be due to reduced density of viable hippocampal neurons. This is consistent with the discovery that stress-related neurohormones such as the glucocorticoids can lead to hippocampal degeneration (Sapolsky 1992).

Whereas morphometric studies have focused on structural hippocampal pathology in PTSD, functional neuroimaging studies have largely implicated abnormal activity patterns involving the amygdala and anterior cingulate cortex, as well as anterior and lateral prefrontal areas (e.g., Broca's area). The first PET symptom-provocation study of PTSD employed a script-driven imagery paradigm to demonstrate brain regions exhibiting differential rCBF in patients with PTSD during a symptomatic versus a nonsymptomatic state (Rauch et al. 1996). Although no comparison group was studied, this experiment implicated the amygdala and right-sided paralimbic structures (including the pregenual region, or "affective division," of the anterior cingulate cortex [ACad]) in mediating the symptoms of PTSD. Moreover, this initial study yielded the unexpected finding of deactivation within Broca's area. More recently, a series of three additional symptom-provocation studies were performed in which comparisons between PTSD and control groups yielded convergent results. Shin and colleagues (1999) studied adult women with childhood sexual abuse–related PTSD and a trauma-exposed control group, using PET CBF methods and the script-driven imagery paradigm. Bremner and colleagues (1999) used PET to study combat veterans with and without PTSD while they were being exposed to combat versus neutral pictures and sounds. Liberzon and colleagues (1999) used SPECT to study veterans with and without PTSD, as well as civilian control subjects, during exposure to combat sounds versus white noise. In these studies, the PTSD cohorts showed attenuated activation within the anterior cingulate cortex (Bremner et al. 1999; Shin et al. 1999), greater activation within the amygdala (Liberzon et al. 1999), and greater deactivations within anterior and lateral cortical areas (Bremner et al. 1999; Shin et al. 1999).

Integrating findings from both preclinical and clinical studies suggests that the circuitry normally responsible for threat assessment is important in the pathophysiology of PTSD (Rauch et al. 1998). Within this circuitry, outlined in Figure 5–2, sensory information pertaining to potential threat is processed by the thalamus and relayed to the amygdala. The amygdala, standing at the center of threat assessment, recruits other key structures in determining the threat response. The anterior paralimbic system is recruited to aid in prioritizing competing streams of information. The hippocampus is activated to encode and access relevant information regarding the context of the potential threat. Reciprocal connections from the amygdala to the thalamus serve as feedback to enhance sensory processing to aid in the evaluation of threat. Other critical reciprocal connections from the hippocampus and ACad provide important feedback to the amygdala to aid in determining the response to threat. The hippocampus provides contextual information based on past experiences and the current situation. The medial frontal cortex (particularly the ACad) provides cortical control over the amygdala to facilitate extinction in the absence of true threat. As outlined earlier, neuroimaging studies in PTSD are reminiscent of animal fear conditioning models and point to three regions within this circuitry that may be dysfunctional: the amygdala, the hippocampus, and the anterior cingulate cortex. Further studies will be necessary to test discrete hypotheses regarding 1) hyperresponsivity of the amygdala, 2) inadequate governance of the amygdala by the ACad, and 3) inadequate contextual information processing by the hippocampus.

Neural Circuitry of Obsessive-Compulsive Disorder

Although categorized among the anxiety disorders in DSM-IV-TR (American Psychiatric Association 2000), current neurobiological and clinical evidence supports a closer association between OCD and an array of disorders commonly referred to as obsessive-compulsive (OC)–spectrum disorders (e.g., Tourette syndrome [TS], trichotillomania, body dysmorphic disorder). Whereas the limbic system and amygdalofugal pathways have been emphasized in neuroanatomic models of panic disorder and PTSD, analogous models of OCD and other OC-spectrum disorders have focused on cortico-striato-thalamo-cortical (CSTC) circuitry.

Within the prefrontal cortex, certain functional subterritories have been identified as particularly relevant in OCD. The ventral prefrontal cortex consists of two functional regions, the posteromedial orbitofrontal cortex (PMOFC), a component of the paralimbic system, and the anterior and lateral orbitofrontal cortex (ALOFC). The PMOFC is

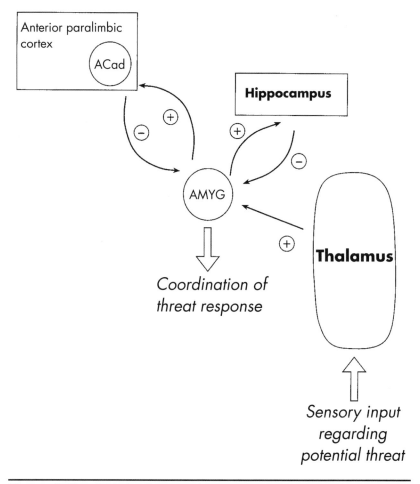

Figure 5–2.   *Critical pathways in threat assessment and response. The amygdala recruits other key structures in determining the threat response. The anterior paralimbic region integrates competing streams of information. The hippocampus encodes and accesses relevant information regarding the context of the potential threat. Reciprocal connections from the amygdala to the thalamus serve as feedback to enhance sensory processing to aid in the evaluation of threat. Other critical reciprocal connections from the hippocampus and the affective division of the anterior cingulate (ACad) provide important feedback to the amygdala to aid in determining the response to threat. The medial frontal cortex (particularly the ACad) provides cortical control over the amygdala to facilitate extinction in the absence of true threat. AMYG = amygdala.*

important in mediating affective and motivational functions (Mesulam 1985). The ALOFC plays the critical intermediary between lateral prefrontal and paralimbic prefrontal areas, controlling response inhibition and behavioral regulation in response to social cues (Mesulam 1985).

Multiple segregated CSTC circuits (Alexander et al. 1986) exist in parallel, each involving projections from specific cortical zones to corresponding subdivisions of the striatum. These projections then connect with the thalamus via other intermediate basal ganglia sites. Finally, these circuits are closed via reciprocal connections from the thalamus back to the same prefrontal cortical regions from which the corticostriatal projections originated. One simple scheme (Alexander et al. 1986) has described four such circuits:

1. The circuit projecting from the sensorimotor cortex to the thalamus via the putamen, subserving sensorimotor functions
2. The circuit projecting from the paralimbic cortex (including the MOFC) to the thalamus via the nucleus accumbens, regulating affective or motivational functions
3. The circuit projecting from the ALOFC to the thalamus via the ventromedial caudate nucleus, mediating context-related functions and response inhibition
4. The circuit projecting from the dorsolateral prefrontal cortex (DLPFC) to the thalamus via the dorsolateral caudate nucleus, subserving working memory and executive functions

Among these four circuits, it is the third, referred to as the *ventral cognitive circuit*, that has been primarily implicated in OCD because of its key interface between the dorsal cognitive and affective systems and its association with response inhibition.

The CSTC circuits contain two major branches that are thought to be relevant to panic disorder and PTSD. These can be viewed as analogous to the declarative (hippocampus) and implicit (amygdala) memory systems described by LeDoux (1996), in that one of them—the cortico-thalamic branch—provides reciprocal communication between the cortex and thalamus that involves consciously accessible input and output streams, and the other—the cortico-striato-thalamic branch—modulates transmission at the thalamus and rapidly processes information without conscious representation (Graybiel 1995). The striatum, therefore, plays the critical role of facilitating information processing at the level of the thalamus by enhancing and filtering input and output, in addition to carrying out certain nonconscious functions. Thus, the striatum may be important in lessening the load on cognitive processing systems, thereby reducing the allocation of precious conscious resources necessary to carry out automatic, rule-based, stereotyped processes (Rauch et al. 1995, 1997a).

Adding to the complexity of the CSTC circuit, each major branch also consists of both a "direct" and an "indirect" pathway (Albin et al. 1989). The net effect of these pathways, operating in parallel, is to oppose influences at the thalamus, as outlined in Figure 5–3. The direct system is defined by its direct projections from the striatum to the globus pallidus interna to the thalamus, where the end effect is excitatory (i.e., "amplifying" thalamic throughput). The indirect system is defined by its indirect projections from the striatum to the globus pallidus interna, involving an intermediary loop from the globus pallidus externa to the subthalamic nucleus to the globus pallidus interna, and then to the thalamus. The net result of this circuit is an inhibitory influence on the thalamus (i.e., "filtering" thalamic throughput).

This complex neuroanatomy provides a framework for understanding current neurobiological models of OCD, which rely on hypotheses involving aberrant functioning within this circuitry. Early models of OCD suggested general excessive, reverberating activity of the cortico-thalamic circuit (Baxter et al. 1990). These models were ultimately revised to incorporate the role of the direct and indirect pathways in balancing activity at the thalamus. Thus, it was proposed that dominance of the direct system in OCD would lead to disinhibition of the thalamus, resulting in overdrive of the cortico-thalamic division (Rauch and Jenike 1993). Investigators also examined more closely the relationship between OCD and TS, and the first theories suggesting that OCD and TS might share a similar pathophysiology were proposed (Baxter et al. 1990). An examination of the possible relationship between the different CSTC circuits and certain clinical symptom phenomena resulted in the so-called striatal topography model of OC-spectrum disorders (Rauch and Jenike 1997). Specifically, dysfunction in the putamen-based circuitry was postulated to be responsible for the sensorimotor symptoms of TS, whereas dysfunction in the ventromedial caudate-based circuitry was proposed for OCD.

Neuroimaging studies in OCD have provided overwhelming evidence of CSTC involvement. Despite negative findings and some inconsistency in results (Aylward et al. 1996), the available literature suggests subtle striatal volumetric abnormalities in OCD (Robinson et al. 1995). Moreover, whereas the caudate has been principally implicated in volumetric studies of OCD, the putamen has been implicated in TS (Singer et al. 1993) as well as in trichotillomania (O'Sullivan et al. 1997). Interestingly, initial MRS studies have likewise found reduced striatal NAA in OCD (Bartha et al. 1998), which is consistent with the notion of a primary pathological lesion within the striatum. Recent data have also

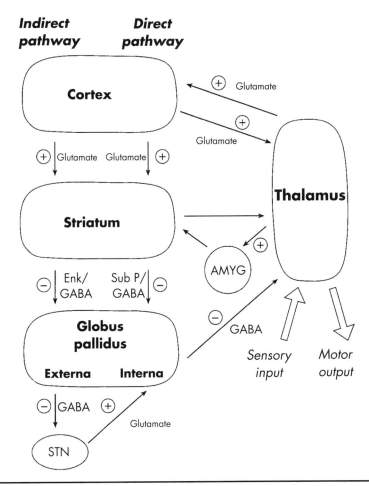

Figure 5–3. *Direct and indirect pathways of the cortico-striato-thalamo-cortical (CSTC) circuit. The cortico-thalamic branch provides reciprocal communication between the cortex and the thalamus that involves consciously accessible input and output streams. The collateral branch, the cortico-striato-thalamic branch, modulates transmission at the thalamus and rapidly processes information without conscious representation. Each major branch also consists of both a "direct" and an "indirect" pathway. The direct system is defined by its direct projections from the striatum to the globus pallidus interna to the thalamus, where the end effect is excitatory. The indirect system is defined by its indirect projections from the striatum to the globus pallidus interna, involving an intermediary loop from the globus pallidus externa to the subthalamic nucleus to the globus pallidus interna, and then to the thalamus. The net result of this circuit is an inhibitory influence on the thalamus. Enk = enkephalin; Sub P = substance P; GABA = γ-aminobutyric acid; AMYG = amygdala; STN = subthalamic nucleus.*

emerged in support of an autoimmune-mediated mechanism of striatal degeneration in precipitous cases of early-onset OCD or TS (Swedo et al. 1998). It should be noted that, in addition to striatal findings, there have been reports of significant white matter reductions in OCD (Breiter et al. 1994), suggesting that OCD may be a consequence of abnormal early brain development in some cases.

Functional imaging studies of OCD provide an even more consistent complement of findings (see Rauch et al. 2001 for review). Studies of OCD patients during a nonsymptomatic state have indicated hyperactivity within the orbitofrontal cortex, the anterior cingulate cortex, and the caudate (see Rauch et al. 2001 for review) that is accentuated with symptom provocation (Breiter et al. 1996; Rauch et al. 1997a) and attenuated with successful treatment (Baxter et al. 1992). Furthermore, the magnitude of pretreatment glucose metabolic rates within the prefrontal cortex predicts response to subsequent treatment. Low levels of metabolism within the orbitofrontal cortex and anterior cingulate cortex predict a good response to serotonin reuptake inhibitors, whereas higher levels of metabolism within the orbitofrontal cortex may predict preferential response to behavioral therapy (Saxena et al. 1998). Cognitive activation paradigms have been developed as reliable and sensitive probes of striato-thalamic function in the context of an implicit information-processing task (see Rauch et al. 1997b). Using this paradigm, Rauch and colleagues have demonstrated deficient striato-thalamic recruitment, as well as aberrant hippocampal activity, in OCD (Rauch et al. 1997b, 2001).

Taken together, these findings support a striatal topography model of OC-spectrum disorders; in particular, OCD appears to be characterized by dysfunction within the orbitofrontal-caudate CSTC circuit. Furthermore, primary striatal pathology is implicated in at least a subset of OCD cases.

Signaling Pathways

Signaling Pathways in Panic Disorder

Several major neurotransmitter systems have been implicated in the pathophysiology of panic disorder, including norepinephrine, serotonin (5-hydroxytryptamine [5-HT]), γ-aminobutyric acid (GABA), and corticotropin-releasing hormone (CRH). Much of the investigation into the function of these systems in panic has used physiological and pharmacological challenges to elicit panic reactions. Among the agents successfully used to evoke panic attacks in panic subjects are sodium lactate, sodium bicarbonate, inhaled carbon dioxide, isoproterenol, doxapram, yohimbine, *m*-chlorophenylpiperazine (mCPP), fenflura-mine, β-carboline, caffeine, and CCK agonists (see Coplan and Klein 1996). The success of such a diverse group of agents in eliciting panic attacks in this population suggests a low threshold for the triggering of panic pathways by a variety of mechanisms.

Studies of norepinephrine neurotransmission in panic disorder have principally relied on pharmacological challenge paradigms using clonidine, an α_2 agonist, and yohimbine, an α_2 antagonist. Challenge with clonidine results in the reliable finding of a blunted growth hormone (GH) response in panic patients (Sullivan et al. 1998), often interpreted as evidence of decreased postsynaptic α_2-adrenergic receptor sensitivity in panic disorder. In panic disorder patients, yohimbine challenge stimulates locus coeruleus firing and norepinephrine release, eliciting high rates of panic accompanied by increases in serum levels of 3-methoxy-4-hydroxyphenylglycol (MHPG), the principal noradrenergic metabolite. Specific adrenergic agonists and the carotid chemoreceptor stimulator doxapram may act in part via peripheral receptors that relay information via vagal and glossopharyngeal afferents to the nucleus tractus solitarius (NTS). The NTS is known to influence the amygdala via projections to the sensory thalamus and the parabrachial nucleus (see Figure 5–1) (Berkley and Scofield 1990).

Studies of serotonin neurotransmission in panic disorder have principally employed the mixed serotonin agonist-antagonist mCPP and the indirect serotonin agonist fenfluramine. Patients with panic disorder have demonstrated increased rates of anxiety, but not necessarily overt panic attacks, in response to these agents (Wetzler et al. 1996). The enhanced responsivity to serotonin-releasing agents raises the possibility of postsynaptic 5-HT hypersensitivity in panic disorder due to chronically depressed serotonergic neurotransmission. Preclinical studies suggest that serotonergic neurons originating in the raphe nuclei modulate an evolved, complex response to threat. A 5-HT pathway originating in the dorsal raphe nucleus (DRN) innervates the amygdala and frontal cortex via the medial forebrain bundle. This pathway is hypothesized to facilitate active escape and avoidance behaviors in response to distal threat (Graeff et al. 1996). It is assumed that these behaviors rely on learning and relate to conditioned or anticipatory anxiety. A DRN pathway innervates the periventricular and PAG region such that 5-HT neurons inhibit inborn flight-or-fight responses to proximal danger, acute pain, or asphyxia. Thus, 5-HT has been implicated as an important modulator within the neurocircuitry of fear responses.

The significance of the GABA-benzodiazepine receptor complex in the mediation of anxiety has been firmly established in the preclinical literature. These findings, along with the established clinical efficacy of benzodiazepines in the treatment of panic disorder (Davidson 1997), have made the GABA system a subject of significant research interest. Plasma studies of GABA levels have demonstrated no differences between panic patients and healthy controls (Roy-Byrne et al. 1992). Pharmacological challenge studies aimed at determining alterations in benzodiazepine receptor sensitivity in panic disorder have produced conflicting results. One group demonstrated anxiogenic effects of flumazenil (a $GABA_A$ antagonist) (Nutt et al. 1990); another group found no significant effect of flumazenil in two later studies (Strohle et al. 1999). Likewise, results of receptor imaging studies in panic disorder have been inconclusive. The earliest studies suggested decreased benzodiazepine binding in the hippocampus and left temporal lobe (Kaschka et al. 1995) and increased benzodiazepine binding in the right prefrontal-temporal cortex (Kuikka et al. 1995). Studies applying more sophisticated quantitative PET receptor technology have recently reported conflicting results regarding alterations in benzodiazepine binding, which may reflect differences in methodology. Using rigorous methods and a well-defined patient population, Malizia and colleagues (1998) observed significant decreases in receptor binding, particularly in the right orbitofrontal and insular cortices. Abadie and colleagues (1999) reported no differences in benzodiazepine binding in a study of a heterogeneous group of patients with various anxiety disorders, including panic. The current weight of imaging evidence therefore suggests decreased benzodiazepine receptor binding in panic disorder.

Evidence for neuroendocrine dysfunction in panic disorder has also been demonstrated in studies of the HPA axis. The α_2 agonist clonidine has been shown to induce greater decreases in serum cortisol in panic patients compared with healthy controls (Coplan et al. 1995). In addition, panic patients demonstrate an uncoupling of the noradrenergic-HPA axis, as evidenced by absence of the typical correlation between MHPG and cortisol, both at baseline and in response to clonidine challenge (Coplan et al. 1997). An analysis of data from sodium lactate studies conducted between 1984 and 1998 found that fear, high cortisol, and low partial pressure of carbon dioxide (pCO_2) during the baseline period (just prior to lactate infusion) were the strongest predictors of panic (Coplan et al. 1998). Such predictors are consistent with amygdalar activation affecting changes in cortical areas (cognitive misappraisal), the paraventricular nucleus of the hypothalamus (HPA axis activation), and the parabrachial nucleus (hyperventilation), respectively.

Signaling Pathways in Posttraumatic Stress Disorder

The critical neural pathways implicated in the pathophysiology of PTSD, as described above, are hypothesized to involve a hypersensitive/hyperresponsive amygdala associated with inadequate governance by the hippocampus and ACad. Although any discussion of neurochemical dysregulation within these specific pathways is preliminary, possible substrates include the catecholamine, 5-HT, and glucocorticoid systems.

Disordered physiological arousal is a key component of PTSD; patients are unable to discriminate between threatening and innocuous stimuli, reacting to neutral stimuli with a degree of arousal in keeping with the original traumatic event. This has been demonstrated repeatedly in studies examining the physiological response of PTSD patients to images and sounds reminiscent of the specific trauma. PTSD subjects respond to these stimuli with significant increases in autonomic and stress-related parameters such as blood pressure, heart rate, and skin conductance (Pitman et al. 1987) and demonstrate an exaggerated startle (Butler et al. 1990). PTSD patients also respond to pharmacological agents that stimulate physiological arousal (e.g., yohimbine and lactate) with affective experiences (images, intrusive thoughts, flashbacks) reflecting the prior trauma (Southwick et al. 1993). Biochemical support for physiological hyperreactivity in terms of increased sympathetic function in PTSD is less consistent. Although an early report suggested the possibility of an abnormal elevation of sympathetic neurotransmission in PTSD (Kosten et al. 1987), most investigators have found normal basal sympathetic activity (McFall et al. 1992).

More definitive abnormalities have been reported in HPA axis functioning in PTSD. On the basis of what is known from preclinical work regarding damaging, stress-related effects of the glucocorticoids on neuronal structures, PTSD patients were expected to display hyperreactivity of the HPA axis. However, contrary to expectations, the first report of HPA axis function in PTSD suggested significant downregulation of the peripheral HPA axis (Yehuda et al. 1990). Yehuda and colleagues demonstrated in a series of studies that PTSD subjects have lower plasma cortisol and 24-hour urinary cortisol excretion. However, Lemieux and Coe (1995) reported higher levels of 24-hour urinary cortisol levels in women with childhood sexual abuse–related PTSD compared with healthy controls. Greater suppression of cortisol, in response to dexamethasone administration, in PTSD subjects has been reported by several research groups (Yehuda et al. 1993). Preclinical models of chronic stress are consistent with these findings, which suggest downregulation of the peripheral system and a loss of cortisol reactivity.

Signaling Pathways in Obsessive-Compulsive Disorder

The two neurotransmitter systems most prominently implicated in the pathogenesis of OCD are 5-HT and dopamine. Indirect measures of 5-HT function have included assays of peripheral receptor binding in blood and cerebrospinal fluid of OCD subjects and pharmacological challenges used to stimulate 5-HT release and examine consequent changes in endocrine or behavioral measures. These studies have yielded inconsistent results and have generally been criticized on the basis of their nonspecific nature. Thus, there is currently little empirical evidence to support a serotonergic hypothesis of OCD pathophysiology. Nonetheless, it is clear that modulation of serotonergic neurotransmission is a key factor in the successful pharmacotherapy of OCD. Although the specific neuropharmacological effects of the selective serotonin reuptake inhibitors (SSRIs) on the frontal cortex and other key areas in OCD are not currently known, preclinical studies confirm that these and other antidepressants potentiate serotonergic transmission (Blier and de Montigny 1994). SSRI-induced therapeutic changes are mediated by the process of autoreceptor desensitization (Blier et al. 1998), which in animal studies has been shown to occur more rapidly in the lateral frontal cortex than in the medial frontal cortex (el Mansari et al. 1995). These data support the idea that the therapeutic effect of the SSRIs in OCD, following a delay of several weeks, involves downregulation of terminal autoreceptors (5-HT$_{1D}$) in the orbitofrontal cortex, thereby facilitating serotonergic transmission in that region. Interestingly, the antidepressant effects of SSRIs, purportedly mediated within the lateral frontal cortex, are also known to occur earlier than their antiobsessional effects. Antiobsessional effects are most likely mediated within the medial frontal (orbitofrontal) cortex. This is also consistent with clinical evidence demonstrating that those OC-spectrum disorders that are believed to involve dysfunction within the cognitive and affective cortico-striatal circuits appear to be preferentially responsive to SSRIs, whereas chronic tics involving sensorimotor CSTC circuits are not.

It is not clear how current information regarding the role of 5-HT in OCD generalizes to other OC-spectrum disorders, such as body dysmorphic disorder, trichotillomania, and TS. Although SSRIs appear to be effective in reducing some of the symptomatology of body dysmorphic disorder and trichotillomania, they are not effective in reducing tics in TS. Dopamine antagonists, however, are effective in reducing tics in TS, a finding consistent with data suggesting a fundamental striatal dopaminergic abnormality in this disorder (Malison et al. 1995). Thus, one possibility is that non-tic-related OCD and body dysmorphic disorders involve pathophysiology of the orbitofrontal-caudate circuitry, whereas tic-related OCD and TS involve primary striatal pathology. Hence, serotonergic modulation at the level of the orbitofrontal cortex may be sufficient for antiobsessional effects in body dysmorphic disorder or non-tic-related OCD, while dopaminergic modulation within the striatum may work synergistically with orbitofrontal serotonergic modulation to relieve tic-related OCD. Finally, pure TS may respond to dopamine modulation at the level of the striatum, without the need for serotonergic modulation in the orbitofrontal cortex.

Psychopharmacology

Psychopharmacology of Panic Disorder

The 5-HT, norepinephrine, and GABA systems have been the traditional targets for modern anxiolytic medications, including the heterocyclic antidepressants, the monoamine oxidase inhibitors (MAOIs), the SSRIs, and the benzodiazepines. The heterocyclic antidepressants, established as among the first medications with powerful antipanic properties (Klein 1964), have gradually been superseded by the advent of newer antidepressants with similar antipanic efficacies and superior side-effect profiles. Likewise, the MAOIs, although clearly established to be effective treatments, have yielded to the newer antidepressants, which have fewer drug-drug and dietary interactions. The high-potency benzodiazepines, particularly alprazolam and clonazepam, remain mainstays of treatment for panic disorder. Both alprazolam and clonazepam have been extensively studied and shown to be effective, well tolerated, and safe in this population (Davidson 1997).

Among the newer classes of antidepressants currently in use for the treatment of panic disorder, the SSRIs have become first-line treatments. The effectiveness of the SSRIs in panic disorder has been established in several large, multicenter, placebo-controlled studies that suggest that these agents ameliorate both the somatic and the psychic symptoms of anxiety (Ballenger et al. 1998; Lepola et al. 1998; Michelson et al. 1998). Although the SSRIs tend to be well tolerated overall, they have certain limitations, including anxiogenic effects at initiation of treatment, delayed onset of anxiolysis, sexual side effects, and weight gain with long-term use. In addition, up to one-third of patients will be nonresponders. Other antidepressants with demonstrated efficacy are the serotonin-norepinephrine reuptake inhibitor (SNRI) venlafaxine (Pollack et al. 1996) and the $5-HT_2$ antagonist and weak SNRI nefazodone (Zajecka

1996). Additional drugs being used in the treatment of panic disorder are the anticonvulsants gabapentin and valproate and long-acting β-blockers such as betaxolol (Baetz and Bowen 1998; Swartz 1998).

Psychopharmacology of Posttraumatic Stress Disorder

As reviewed earlier, the symptomatology of PTSD is broader than that of the other anxiety disorders, and therefore pharmacological treatment must address a wide array of symptoms, including intrusive thoughts/ images; numbing, withdrawal, and avoidance; physiological arousal; depression; and sleep disturbances. Because no single medication is effective in targeting all PTSD symptoms, multiple medications and psychotherapy or behavioral treatment are often incorporated in the treatment of PTSD.

Several classes of medications have been shown to be effective in the treatment of uncomplicated PTSD, including the tricyclics (Kosten et al. 1991) and the MAOIs (Frank et al. 1988). Although the benzodiazepines are frequently prescribed as adjunctive treatments in this disorder, particularly for their sleep benefits, they have not been shown to be effective as a primary treatment (Braun et al. 1990). At present, the SSRIs are probably the most widely prescribed agents for the treatment of PTSD, although evidence for their efficacy is based primarily on case studies and open series (see Kent et al. 1998) and a single double-blind, placebo-controlled study (van der Kolk et al. 1994).

Because sympathetic arousal and hyperreactivity are so prominent in PTSD, several investigators have examined the use of mood stabilizers based on the theory that these agents may reduce stress-activated limbic system kindling. Early reports from open trials suggest that valproate may be useful in treatment, particularly for symptoms of hyperarousal (Fesler 1991). Among the newer antidepressants, nefazodone, a novel antidepressant with 5-HT$_2$ antagonist activity and weak serotonin-norepinephrine reuptake inhibition, has attracted interest. Nefazodone has demonstrated promise in several open trials in PTSD and may be particularly useful in repairing sleep disturbances, in addition to ameliorating other PTSD symptoms (Hidalgo et al. 1999).

Psychopharmacology of Obsessive-Compulsive Disorder

The majority of OCD patients respond only partially to pharmacotherapy; therefore, an integrative treatment approach that includes behavioral therapy significantly increases the likelihood of therapeutic success. The pharmacological agents used successfully in the treatment of pure OCD all have in common the feature of 5-HT reuptake inhibition (Jefferson and Greist 1996). Clomipramine, a heterocyclic antidepressant with significant 5-HT reuptake inhibition properties and with well-established efficacy, has been a first-line agent in the treatment of OCD since the early 1990s (Clomipramine Collaborative Study Group 1991). The SSRIs are also well established as effective treatments for OCD (Rasmussen et al. 1997). SSRIs are often a first-choice treatment (before clomipramine) because of their better tolerability.

Augmentation for partial responders has been attempted using numerous agents, with limited success. Behavioral treatment, which should include exposure and response prevention, should always be the first choice for adjunctive treatment. Pharmacological agents that have been used with some success for SSRI/clomipramine augmentation include 5-HT–enhancing agents (e.g., buspirone, fenfluramine), dopamine-blocking agents (e.g., risperidone, haloperidol, pimozide), and benzodiazepines (e.g., clonazepam). As discussed earlier in this chapter, the heterogeneity of OCD itself and of the OC-spectrum disorders may explain why some subtypes are responsive to SSRIs alone, other subtypes are responsive to SSRIs with the addition of a dopamine antagonist, and still others are unresponsive to either of these strategies. For OCD patients who have a poor response to the standard treatments described above, options include intravenous administration of clomipramine and, in extreme cases, neurosurgery aimed at disrupting CSTC pathways (capsulotomy, cingulotomy).

Advances in neurocircuitry, neurochemistry, and pharmacology are beginning to converge into more detailed and complete models of anxiety. Neuroimaging studies suggest that the anxiety disorders share certain mediating structures, such as the anterior paralimbic cortex, sensory cortex, amygdala, hippocampus, and striatum. However, imaging techniques have also provided data supporting patterns of dysfunction in specific brain regions that distinguish the individual anxiety disorders. For instance, paralimbic dysfunction and lack of appropriate frontal cortex recruitment have been suggested in panic disorder, amygdalar hyperactivity and anterior cingulate dysfunction have been implicated in PTSD, and dysfunction within orbitofrontal-caudate pathways has been demonstrated in OCD.

Conclusions

As our understanding of the neurochemistry of the anxiety disorders continues to grow, so also does the need to understand the roles of signaling pathways on these identified circuits. In concert with functional neuroimaging, experiments involving pharmacological manipulations should provide further clues about the role of specific neurotransmitters within these circuits. The continued development of new radioligands for receptor neuroimaging holds tremendous promise for furthering our understanding both of the complexities of the neurotransmitter systems and of how effective antianxiety medications influence these systems.

Thus, as pathophysiological models of the anxiety disorders continue to evolve, the need to integrate findings from structural, functional, and neuroreceptor imaging studies with information gained from preclinical, clinical, and genetic studies is paramount. Only through this type of integrative approach will treatments become more sophisticated and targeted, thereby providing better options for patients with anxiety disorders.

References

Abadie P, Boulenger JP, Benali K, et al: Relationships between trait and state anxiety and the central benzodiazepine receptor: a PET study. Eur J Neurosci 11:1470–1478, 1999

Adolphs R, Tranel D, Damasio H, et al: Impaired recognition of emotion in facial expressions following bilateral damage to the human amygdala. Nature 372:669–672, 1994

Albin RL, Young AB, Penny JB: The functional anatomy of basal ganglia disorders. Trends Neurosci 12:366–375, 1989

Alexander GE, DeLong MR, Strick PL: Parallel organization of functionally segregated circuits linking basal ganglia and cortex. Annu Rev Neurosci 9: 357–381, 1986

Aylward EH, Harris GJ, Hoehn-Saric R, et al: Normal caudate nucleus in obsessive-compulsive disorder assessed by quantitative neuroimaging. Arch Gen Psychiatry 53:577–584, 1996

American Psychiatric Association: Diagnostic and Statistical Manual of Mental Disorders, 4th Edition, Text Revision. Washington, DC, American Psychiatric Association, 2000

Baetz M, Bowen RC: Efficacy of divalproex sodium in patients with panic disorder and mood instability who have not responded to conventional therapy. Can J Psychiatry 43:73–77, 1998

Ballenger JC, Wheadon DE, Steiner M, et al: Double-blind, fixed-dose, placebo-controlled study of paroxetine in the treatment of panic disorder. Am J Psychiatry 155:36–42, 1998

Bartha R, Stein MB, Williamson PC, et al: A short echo 1H spectroscopy and volumetric MRI study of the corpus striatum in patients with obsessive-compulsive disorder and comparison subjects. Am J Psychiatry 155:1584–1591, 1998

Baxter LR Jr, Schwartz JM, Guze BH, et al: Neuroimaging in obsessive-compulsive disorder: seeking the mediating neuroanatomy, in Obsessive-Compulsive Disorders: Theory and Management. Edited by Jenike MA, Baer L. Chicago, IL, Year Book Medical, 1990, pp 167–188

Baxter LR Jr, Schwartz JM, Bergman KS, et al: Caudate glucose metabolic rate changes with both drug and behavior therapy for obsessive-compulsive disorder. Arch Gen Psychiatry 49:681–689, 1992

Bechara A, Tranel D, Damasio H, et al: Double dissociation of conditioning and declarative knowledge relative to the amygdala and hippocampus in humans. Science 269:1115–1118, 1995

Berkley KJ, Scofield SL: Relays from the spinal cord and solitary nucleus through the parabrachial nucleus to the forebrain in the cat. Brain Res 529:333–338, 1990

Blier P, de Montigny C: Current advances and trends in the treatment of depression. Trends Pharmacol Sci 15:220–226, 1994

Blier P, Pineyro G, el Mansari M, et al: Role of somatodendritic 5-HT autoreceptors in modulating 5-HT neurotransmission. Ann N Y Acad Sci 861:204–216, 1998

Braun P, Greenberg B, Basperg H, et al: Core symptoms of posttraumatic stress disorder unimproved by alprazolam treatment. J Clin Psychiatry 51:236–238, 1990

Breiter HC, Filipek PA, Kennedy DN, et al: Retrocallosal white matter abnormalities in patients with obsessive compulsive disorder. Arch Gen Psychiatry 51:663–663, 1994

Breiter HC, Rauch SL, Kwong KK, et al: Functional magnetic resonance imaging of symptom provocation in obsessive compulsive disorder. Arch Gen Psychiatry 53:595–606, 1996

Bremner JD, Randall P, Scott TM, et al: MRI-based measurement of hippocampal volume in patients with combat-related posttraumatic stress disorder. Am J Psychiatry 152:973–981, 1995

Bremner JD, Staib LH, Kaloupek D, et al: Neural correlates of exposure to traumatic pictures and sound in Vietnam combat veterans with and without posttraumatic stress disorder: a positron emission tomography study. Biol Psychiatry 45:806–816, 1999

Butler R, Braff D, Rausch J, et al: Physiological evidence of exaggerated startle response in a subgroup of Vietnam veterans with combat-related posttraumatic stress disorder. Am J Psychiatry 147:1308–1312, 1990

Cedarbaum JM, Aghajanian GK: Afferent projections to the rat locus coeruleus as determined by a retrograde tracing technique. J Comp Neurol 178:1–16, 1978

Clomipramine Collaborative Study Group: Clomipramine in the treatment of patients with obsessive-compulsive disorder. Arch Gen Psychiatry 48:730–738, 1991

Coplan JD, Klein DF: Pharmacologic probes in panic disorder, in Advances in the Neurobiology of Anxiety Disorders. Edited by Westenberg HGM, den Boer JA, Murphy DL. New York, Wiley, 1996, pp 179–204

Coplan JD, Pine D, Papp L, et al: Uncoupling of the noradrenergic-hypothalamic-pituitary-adrenal axis in panic disorder. Neuropsychopharmacology 13:65–73, 1995

Coplan JD, Papp LA, Pine D, et al: Clinical improvement with fluoxetine therapy and noradrenergic function in patients with panic disorder. Arch Gen Psychiatry 54:643–648, 1997

Coplan JD, Goetz R, Klein DF, et al: Plasma cortisol concentrations preceding lactate-induced panic. Psychological, biochemical, and physiological correlates. Arch Gen Psychiatry 55:130–136, 1998

Davidson JR: Use of benzodiazepines in panic disorder. J Clin Psychiatry 58 (suppl 2):26–28, 1997

Davis M: The role of the amygdala in fear and anxiety. Annu Rev Neurosci 15: 353–375, 1992

De Oca BM, DeCola JP, Maren S, et al: Distinct regions of the periaqueductal gray are involved in the acquisition and expression of defensive responses. J Neurosci 18:3426–3432, 1998

de Olmos JS: Amygdaloid nuclear gray complex, in The Human Nervous System. Edited by Paxinos GT. San Diego, CA, Academic Press, 1990, pp 583–710

Dunn JD, Whitener J: Plasma corticosterone responses to electrical stimulation of the amygdaloid complex: cytoarchitectural specificity. Neuroendocrinology 42:211–217, 1986

el Mansari M, Bouchard C, Blier P: Alteration of serotonin release in the guinea pig orbito-frontal cortex by selective serotonin reuptake inhibitors: relevance to treatment of obsessive-compulsive disorder. Neuropsychopharmacology 13:117–127, 1995

Fesler FA: Valproate in combat-related posttraumatic stress disorder. J Clin Psychiatry 52:361–364, 1991

Frank JB, Kosten TR, Giller EL Jr, et al: A randomized clinical trial of phenelzine and imipramine for posttraumatic stress disorder. Am J Psychiatry 145: 1289–1291, 1988

Graeff FG, Guimaraes FS, De Andrade TG, et al: Role of 5-HT in stress, anxiety, and depression. Pharmacol Biochem Behav 54:129–141, 1996

Graybiel AM: Building action repertoires: memory and learning functions of the basal ganglia. Curr Opin Neurobiol 5:733–741, 1995

Halgren E, Walter RD, Cherlow DG, et al: Mental phenomena evoked by electrical stimulation of the human hippocampal formation and amygdala. Brain 101:83–117, 1978

Hidalgo R, Hertzberg MA, Mellman T, et al: Nefazodone in post-traumatic stress disorder: results from six open-label trials. Int Clin Psychopharmacol 14:61–68, 1999

Javanmard M, Shlik J, Kennedy SH, et al: Neuroanatomic correlates of CCK-4-induced panic attacks in healthy humans: a comparison of two time points. Biol Psychiatry 45:872–882, 1999

Jefferson JW, Greist JH: The pharmacotherapy of obsessive-compulsive disorder. Psychiatric Annals 26:202–209, 1996

Kaschka W, Feistel H, Ebert D: Reduced benzodiazepine receptor binding in panic disorders measured by iomazenil SPECT. J Psychiatr Res 29:427–434, 1995

Kent JM, Coplan JD, Gorman JM: Clinical utility of the selective serotonin reuptake inhibitors in the spectrum of anxiety. Biol Psychiatry 44:812–824, 1998

Ketter TA, Andreason PJ, George MS, et al: Anterior paralimbic mediation of procaine-induced emotional and psychosensory experiences. Arch Gen Psychiatry 53:59–69, 1996

Kim JJ, Fanselow MS: Modality-specific retrograde amnesia of fear. Science 256: 675–677, 1992

Klein DF: Delineation of two drug responses for anxiety syndromes. Psychopharmacologia 5:397–408, 1964

Kosten TR, Mason JW, Giller EL, et al: Sustained urinary norepinephrine and epinephrine elevation in post-traumatic stress disorder. Psychoneuroendocrinology 12:13–20, 1987

Kosten TR, Frank JB, Dan E, et al: Pharmacotherapy for post-traumatic stress disorder using phenelzine or imipramine. J Nerv Ment Dis 179:366–370, 1991

Kuikka JT, Pitkanen A, Lepola U, et al: Abnormal regional benzodiazepine receptor uptake in the prefrontal cortex in patients with panic disorder. Nucl Med Comm 16:273–280, 1995

LaBar KS, Gatenby JC, Gore JC, et al: Human amygdala activation during conditioned fear acquisition and extinction: a mixed-trial fMRI study. Neuron 20:937–945, 1998

LeDoux JE: The Emotional Brain. New York, Simon & Schuster, 1996

LeDoux JE, Iwata J, Cicchetti P, et al: Different projections of the central amygdaloid nucleus mediate autonomic and behavioral correlates of conditioned fear. J Neurosci 8:2517–2519, 1988

LeDoux JE, Cicchetti P, Xagoraris A, et al: The lateral amygdaloid nucleus: sensory interface of the amygdala in fear conditioning. J Neurosci 10:1062–1069, 1990

Lemieux AM, Coe CL: Abuse-related posttraumatic stress disorder: evidence for chronic neuroendocrine activation in women. Psychosom Med 57:105–115, 1995

Lepola UM, Wade AG, Leinonen EV, et al: A controlled, prospective, 1-year trial of citalopram in the treatment of panic disorder. J Clin Psychiatry 59:528–534, 1998

Liberzon I, Taylor SF, Amdur R, et al: Brain activation in PTSD in response to trauma-related stimuli. Biol Psychiatry 45:817–826, 1999

Majidishad P, Pelli DG, LeDoux JE: Disruption of fear conditioning to contextual stimuli but not to a tone by lesions of the accessory basal nucleus of the amygdala. Society for Neuroscience Abstracts 22:1116, 1996

Malison RT, McDougle CJ, van Dyck CH, et al: [123I]beta-CIT SPECT imaging of striatal dopamine transporter binding in Tourette's disorder. Am J Psychiatry 152:1359–1361, 1995

Malizia AL, Cunningham VJ, Bell CJ, et al: Decreased brain GABA(A)-benzodiazepine receptor binding in panic disorder: preliminary results from a quantitative PET study. Arch Gen Psychiatry 55:715–720, 1998

McFall ME, Veith RC, Murburg MM: Basal sympathoadrenal function in posttraumatic stress disorder. Biol Psychiatry 31:1051–1056, 1992

Mesulam M-M: Patterns in behavioral neuroanatomy: association areas, the limbic system, and hemispheric specialization, in Principles of Behavioral Neurology. Edited by Mesulam M-M. Philadelphia, PA, FA Davis, 1985, pp 1–70

Michelson D, Lydiard RB, Pollack MH, et al: Outcome assessment and clinical improvement in panic disorder: evidence from a randomized controlled trial of fluoxetine and placebo. The Fluoxetine Panic Disorder Study Group. Am J Psychiatry 155:1570–1577, 1998

Nutt DJ, Glue P, Lawson C, et al: Flumazenil provocation of panic attacks: evidence for altered benzodiazepine receptor sensitivity in panic disorder. Arch Gen Psychiatry 47:917–925, 1990

O'Sullivan RL, Rauch SL, Breiter HC, et al: Reduced basal ganglia volumes in trichotillomania measured via morphometric magnetic resonance imaging. Biol Psychiatry 42:39–45, 1997

Pitman RK, Orr SP, Forgue DF, et al: Psychophysiologic assessment of posttraumatic stress disorder imagery in Vietnam combat veterans. Arch Gen Psychiatry 44:970–975, 1987

Pollack MH, Worthington JJ 3rd, Ott MW, et al: Venlafaxine for panic disorder: results from a double-blind, placebo-controlled study. Psychopharmacol Bull 32:667–670, 1996

Price JL, Amaral DG: An autoradiographic study of the projections of the central nucleus of the monkey amygdala. J Neurosci 1:1242–1259, 1981

Rasmussen S, Hackett E, DuBoff E, et al: A 2-year study of sertraline in the treatment of obsessive-compulsive disorder. Int Clin Psychopharmacol 12:309–316, 1997

Rauch SL, Jenike MA: Neurobiological models of obsessive-compulsive disorder. Psychosomatics 34:20–32, 1993

Rauch SL, Jenike MA: Neural mechanisms of obsessive-compulsive disorder. Current Review of Mood and Anxiety Disorders 1:84–94, 1997

Rauch SL, Savage CR, Brown HD, et al: A PET investigation of implicit and explicit sequence learning. Human Brain Mapping 3:271–286, 1995

Rauch SL, van der Kolk BA, Fisler RE, et al: A symptom provocation study of posttraumatic stress disorder using positron emission tomography and script-driven imagery. Arch Gen Psychiatry 53:380–387, 1996

Rauch SL, Savage CR, Alpert NM, et al: The functional neuroanatomy of anxiety: a study of three disorders using positron emission tomography and symptom provocation. Biol Psychiatry 42:446–452, 1997a

Rauch SL, Savage CR, Alpert NM, et al: Probing striatal function in obsessive compulsive disorder: a PET study of implicit sequence learning. J Neuropsychiatry Clin Neurosci 9:568–573, 1997b

Rauch SL, Shin LM, Whalen PJ, et al: Neuroimaging and the neuroanatomy of posttraumatic stress disorder. CNS Spectrums 3 (suppl 2):30–41, 1998

Rauch SL, Whalen PJ, Curran T, et al: Probing striato-thalamic function in OCD and TS using neuroimaging methods. Adv Neurol 85:207–224, 2001

Reiman EM, Raichle ME, Butler FK, et al: A focal brain abnormality in panic disorder, a severe form of anxiety. Nature 310:683–685, 1984

Reiman EM, Raichle ME, Robins E, et al: Neuroanatomical correlates of a lactate-induced anxiety attack. Arch Gen Psychiatry 46:493–500, 1989

Robinson D, Wu H, Munne RA, et al: Reduced caudate nucleus volume in obsessive-compulsive disorder. Arch Gen Psychiatry 52:393–398, 1995

Roy-Byrne PP, Cowley DS, Hommer D, et al: Effect of acute and chronic benzodiazepines on plasma GABA in anxious patients and controls. Psychopharmacology (Berl) 109:153–156, 1992

Sapolsky RM: Stress, the Aging Brain, and the Mechanisms of Neuron Death. Cambridge, MA, MIT Press, 1992

Saxena S, Brody AL, Schwartz JM, et al: Neuroimaging and frontal-subcortical circuitry in obsessive-compulsive disorder. Br J Psychiatry 173 (suppl 35): 26–37, 1998

Schuff N, Marmar CR, Weiss DS, et al: Reduced hippocampal volume and N-acetyl aspartate in posttraumatic stress disorder. Ann N Y Acad Sci 821: 516–520, 1997

Shin LM, McNally RJ, Kosslyn SM, et al: Regional cerebral blood flow during script-driven imagery in childhood sexual abuse-related PTSD: a PET investigation. Am J Psychiatry 156:575–584, 1999

Singer HS, Reiss AL, Brown JE, et al: Volumetric MRI changes in basal ganglia of children with Tourette's syndrome. Neurology 43:950–956, 1993

Southwick SM, Krystal JH, Morgan CA, et al: Abnormal noradrenergic function in post traumatic stress disorder. Arch Gen Psychiatry 50:266–274, 1993

Stewart RS, Devous MD Sr, Rush AJ, et al: Cerebral blood flow changes during sodium-lactate-induced panic attacks. Am J Psychiatry 145:442–449, 1988

Strohle A, Kellner M, Holsboer F, et al: Behavioral, neuroendocrine, and cardio-vascular response to flumazenil: no evidence for an altered benzodiazepine receptor sensitivity in panic disorder. Biol Psychiatry 45:321–326, 1999

Sullivan GM, Coplan JD, Gorman JM: Psychoneuroendocrinology of anxiety disorders. Psychiatr Clin North Am 21:397–412, 1998

Swartz CM: Betaxolol in anxiety disorders. Ann Clin Psychiatry 10:9–14, 1998

Swedo SE, Leonard HL, Garvey M, et al: Pediatric autoimmune neuropsychiat-ric disorders associated with streptococcal infections: clinical description of the first 50 cases. Am J Psychiatry 155:264–271, 1998

Takeuchi Y, McLean JH, Hopkins DA: Reciprocal connections between the amygdala and parabrachial nuclei: ultrastructural demonstration by de-generation and axonal transport of horseradish peroxidase in the cat. Brain Res 239:538–588, 1982

van der Kolk BA, Dreyfuss D, Michaels M, et al: Fluoxetine in posttraumatic stress disorder. J Clin Psychiatry 55:517–522, 1994

Wetzler S, Asnis GM, DeLecuona JM, et al: Serotonin function in panic disorder: intravenous administration of meta-chlorophenylpiperazine. Psychiatry Res 62:77–82, 1996

Whalen PJ, Rauch SL, Etcoff NL, et al: Masked presentations of emotional facial expressions modulate amygdala activity without explicit knowledge. J Neurosci 18:411–418, 1998

Yehuda R, Southwick SM, Nussbaum G, et al: Low urinary cortisol excretion in patients with posttraumatic stress disorder. J Nerv Ment Dis 178:366–369, 1990

Yehuda R, Southwick SM, Krystal JH, et al: Enhanced suppression of cortisol following dexamethasone administration in posttraumatic stress disorder. Am J Psychiatry 150:83–86, 1993

Zajecka JM: The effect of nefazodone on comorbid anxiety symptoms associated with depression: experience in family practice and psychiatric outpatient settings. J Clin Psychiatry 57 (suppl 2):10–14, 1996

CHAPTER 6

Neural Circuitry and Signaling in Depression

Gerard Marek, M.D., Ph.D.
Ronald S. Duman, Ph.D.

Clinical Presentation

A wide variety of depressive disorders are currently codified under a number of different diagnostic categories in the *Diagnostic and Statistical Manual of Mental Disorders,* Fourth Edition (DSM-IV; American Psychiatric Association 1994) and its text revision (DSM-IV-TR; American Psychiatric Association 2000). Our understanding of the utility of animal models and antidepressant screens—as well as the pathophysiology and treatment of these various depressive disorders—rests on whether these disorders represent separate illnesses or differing clinical presentations of the same illness.

Major depression is phenomenologically characterized by alterations in mood, neurovegetative signs, and cognition lasting on a daily basis for at least 2 weeks that is not due to a drug of abuse, a medication, or a general medical condition such as hyperthyroidism. Changes in mood include depressed mood (or irritable mood in children and adolescents) and anhedonia. Neurovegetative signs include changes in weight or appetite, insomnia or hypersomnia, psychomotor agitation or retardation, and fatigue. Cognitive features include thoughts of worthlessness or inappropriate guilt, decreased concentration, and recurrent thoughts of suicide.

Major depression may also present with psychotic features that are mood-congruent (e.g., hallucinations and delusions that deal with personal guilt, death, and deserved punishment) or mood-incongruent (e.g., hallucinations and delusions of persecution, thought insertion, thought broadcasting). Patients with major depression with psychotic features have an increased likelihood of suicide and are more likely to have nonsuppression on the dexamethasone suppression test. These patients often have greater psychosomatic complaints, and they appear "physically" sick. Either electroconvulsive therapy (ECT) or a combination of an antidepressant and an antipsychotic drug is the treatment of choice for these patients. Again, it is not clear if depression with psychosis represents the extreme end of major depression with respect to severity or constitutes a separate disorder.

In addition, a number of other depressive syndromes with differing durations and intensities of symptoms are known. Dysthymia is a depressive disorder with symptoms that do not satisfy full criteria for a major depressive episode but that last more than 2 years. Sometimes patients are said to suffer from "double depression," in which patients with dysthymic disorder have an increase in their symptoms that now satisfy criteria for major depression. Several other depressive subtypes occur, such as minor depressive disorder, recurrent brief depression, and subsyndromal symptoms. All of these clinical presentations together with major depression may represent a single illness (Judd 1997). On the other hand, some have argued that major depression is an etiologically heterogeneous disease (Winokur 1997).

The depressive disorders described above are termed unipolar depressive disorders when they are restricted to depressive symptoms. However, about 10% of patients who experience single or multiple episodes of major depression may go on to have a manic episode, characterized by grandiose or expansive mood, decreased need for sleep, pressured speech, racing thoughts, an increase in goal-directed activity, and commission of sexual or financial indiscretions. These patients have *bipolar disorder* (formerly called *manic-depressive disorder*), which is genetically distinct from unipolar major depression (Goodwin and Jamison 1990) (see Chapter 7 in this volume).

Although major depression can be limited to a single episode that may last a few months, it more often constitutes a chronic, lifelong illness, with the risk for repeated episodes approaching 80%. Typical episodes last 5 to 6 months, and most patients experience about four episodes over the course of their lives (Judd 1997). There is increasing concern that each depressive episode may further contribute to the likelihood of future episodes or render treatments inadequate. In the following description of the neurocircuitry of depressive disorders, we discuss evidence of structural as well as functional changes in depressed patients.

Neural Circuitry

Both structural and functional neuroimaging studies have provided evidence for involvement of highly interconnected cortical and limbic structures—such as the prefrontal cortex, medial thalamus, amygdala, ventral striatum, hippocampus, and hypothalamic-pituitary-adrenal (HPA) axis—in unipolar major depression (Figure 6–1).

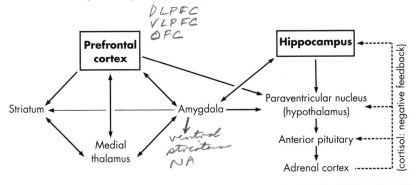

Figure 6–1. *Neuroanatomic circuits with structural and functional alterations as determined by imaging studies done in patients with major depression. The prefrontal cortex and hippocampus are highlighted because recent neuroimaging studies have found evidence of atrophy in these limbic cortical structures. On the **left side** of the figure, extensively interconnected cortical-thalamo-striatal and cortical-thalamo-amygdalar circuits are shown. The **thin line** directed toward the striatum from the amygdala represents the relatively sparse projections to the striatum from the amygdala except for the more robust projections to the ventral striatum (e.g., nucleus accumbens). The **right** side of the figure depicts the hypothalamic-pituitary-adrenal (HPA) axis together with the known influences on the HPA axis by the hippocampus, amygdala, and prefrontal cortex (anterior cingulate). Not shown in the figure is the monoaminergic innervation of these regions by the raphe nuclei, locus coeruleus, and ventral tegmental area.*

Prefrontal Cortex and Major Depression

In particular, a number of structural neuroimaging studies have implicated several cortical areas in major depression. Several different meta-analyses have suggested that ventricular enlargement and cortical sulcal prominence are found in mood disorders (Elkis et al. 1995; Raz and Raz 1990). A magnetic resonance imaging (MRI) study in a group of severely depressed patients referred for ECT found that the volume of the prefrontal cortex was decreased by 7% prior to treatment compared to a group of healthy control subjects (Coffey et al. 1993).

The anatomic specificity of these deficits has been highlighted by results from a positron-emission tomography (PET) study of patients with familial bipolar depression and familial unipolar depression (Drevets et al. 1997). In this study, patients were found to have decreased blood flow in the subgenual prefrontal cortex, an area that mediates emotional and autonomic responses to significant social or provocative stimuli. MRI of the subgenual prefrontal cortex suggested that blood flow was secondary to 39%–48% decreases in the mean gray matter volume of this localized anterior cingulate area. A subsequent study demonstrated that the reduction in the volume of the subgenual prefrontal cortex (Brodmann area 24) is associated with a reduction in the number of glial cells, but not neurons, in this portion of the anterior cingulate (Ongur et al. 1998). This area has extensive connections with structures implicated in emotional behavior and autonomic/neuroendocrine responses to stressors, such as the amygdala, the medial thalamus, the ventral striatum (*i.e.*, the nucleus accumbens), the lateral hypothalamus, and monoaminergic nuclei projecting throughout the neuroaxis.

The histopathology of major depression has been further expanded to include alterations in both neurons and glia in different areas of the prefrontal cortex (Rajkowska et al. 1999). This study used modern computer-assisted three-dimensional cell counting to demonstrate decreases in neuronal size and in both neuronal and glial density in discrete laminae of the rostral orbitofrontal cortex, the ventral orbitofrontal cortex, and the dorsolateral prefrontal cortex. Slightly different changes were seen in the various prefrontal areas that were assessed. These changes also appeared to be present in several patients who had not been exposed to antidepressant drugs.

A number of functional neuroimaging studies have suggested that the blood flow and metabolism in various prefrontal cortical regions may be differentially altered in major depression (see Drevets 1998). Prior to treatment, patients with major depression have reduced glucose metabolism and blood flow in the left dorsolateral and dorsomedial prefrontal cortex (Baxter et al. 1989; Bench et al. 1992; Biver et al. 1994; Bonne et al. 1996). Several (Baxter et al. 1989; Bonne et al. 1996) but not all (Nobler et al. 1994) studies have found that these changes normalize following effective treatment. Bremner et al. (1997) reported that recurrence of depressive symptoms induced by a tryptophan-depletion protocol decreased metabolism in the dorsolateral prefrontal cortex, consistent with the notion that decreased metabolism is associated with the depressive state. Another PET metabolism study found that nonresponders to antidepressant drug therapy showed hypometabolism of the rostral anterior cingulate, whereas antidepressant drug responders displayed a hypermetabolic response (Mayberg et al. 1997).

In contrast to these reports, Drevets et al. (1992, 1997) observed increased blood flow in the left ventrolateral and lateral orbital cortex as well as the medial orbital cortex bilaterally in a group of patients with familial depressive disease. Several other studies provide some support for these findings (Baxter et al. 1989; Buchsbaum et al. 1986). Although the divergent results in the dorsolateral prefrontal cortex and the orbital cortex may appear contradictory, they may be related to the well-established finding, in neuroimaging of various emotional and cognitive processing tasks, of distinct patterns of increases and decreases in cortical blood flow during performance of any given task. For example, similar patterns of increases and decreases in metabolism in different prefrontal regions have been observed during studies of induced sadness in healthy control subjects (Mayberg 1997). Analogous patterns may exist for pathological mood changes such that increases and decreases in metabolism and blood flow may occur simultaneously in different prefrontal regions.

Subcortical Alterations in Major Depression

The prefrontal cortex is well known to be extensively interconnected with the medial thalamus, the amygdala, and the ventral striatum (nucleus accumbens and ventromedial caudate; see Figure 6–1). Functional neuroimaging studies suggest that these areas may be altered in major depression in a manner consistent with findings in the prefrontal cortex. For example, the amygdala is known to share extensive excitatory connections with the ventrolateral and lateral prefrontal cortex as well as with the medial orbital cortex. Blood flow and metabolism in the amygdala has been found to be increased in depression (Abercrombie et al. 1998; Drevets et al. 1992, 1997). Furthermore, the elevated blood flow in the amygdala of depressed patients may be a trait-dependent rather than a state-dependent finding, given that this change remains following remission of depressive symptoms (Drevets et al. 1992). Another study observed increased metabolism in the neocortex and several limbic structures (e.g., amygdala, hippocampus) during the first non–rapid eye movement (REM) period of sleep in depressed patients (Ho et al. 1996). Preliminary observations also suggest that blood flow may be increased in the left medial thalamus in depressed patients (Drevets et al. 1992). Furthermore, decreased brain metabolism in the thalamus, middle frontal gyrus, and orbitofrontal cortex was correlated with increased depressive ratings in remitted depressed patients who experienced a brief (~1 day) return of depressive symptoms following a tryptophan depletion protocol (Bremner et al. 1997).

Finally, the caudate and nucleus accumbens, which are known to receive excitatory connections from the prefrontal cortex, the medial thalamus, and the amygdala, show reduced metabolism and blood flow bilaterally in depressed subjects (Baxter et al. 1985; Drevets et al. 1992). Several MRI studies in primary major depression have suggested that depression is associated with decreased size of the caudate and putamen (Husain et al. 1991; Krishnan et al. 1992). Additional evidence that depression involves circuits including both the prefrontal cortex and the basal ganglia is found in the increased incidence of major depression observed in patients with left-frontal cortical or left-sided basal ganglia strokes, Parkinson's disease, and Huntington's disease (see Cummings 1993).

Hippocampus and HPA Axis

The hippocampus is another limbic cortical area that structural neuro-imaging studies suggest is involved in depression. Hippocampal volume appears to be decreased bilaterally in subjects with a history of depression but currently in clinical remission (Sheline et al. 1996). Furthermore, the decrease in hippocampal volume was correlated with the total duration of symptomatic depressive illness. These results were replicated by Bremner and colleagues (2000). The possibility that the reductions in hippocampal volume can be reversed with long-term antidepressant treatment is also being examined. However, whether these results are related to major depression or are the consequence of stress-induced changes is an open question, given that similar findings have been observed in patients with posttraumatic stress disorder (Bremner et al. 1995; Gurvits et al. 1996) and Cushing's syndrome (Starkman et al. 1992).

Nonetheless, the hippocampal findings are of particular interest, because stress and glucocorticoid administration appear to cause atrophy and suppress neurogenesis in the hippocampus (see McEwen 1999; Sapolsky 1996) (Figure 6–2). Furthermore, the hippocampus may play a role in the dysregulation in fast-feedback control of cortisol secretion observed in depressed patients (Young et al. 1991). In fact, several studies have found structural evidence for changes in the HPA axis, such as increased size of both the pituitary (Krishnan et al. 1991) and the adrenal gland (Nemeroff et al. 1992), in depressed patients. These findings are consistent with the alterations in the function of the HPA axis known to occur in major depression (e.g., hypercortisolism and failure of dexamethasone to suppress cortisol levels). However, it should be remembered that considerable variability for dysregulation of the HPA axis exists in individual depressed patients, depending on the clinical presentation (e.g., psychotic vs. nonpsychotic, melancholic vs. nonmelancholic) (Nelson and Davis 1997). Again, it is not clear whether this variability reflects differing severity or different subtypes of mood disorder.

Cellular and Molecular Determinants of Stress and Depression

The underlying pathophysiology of depression most likely involves the dysregulation of multiple endocrine and neurotransmitter systems.

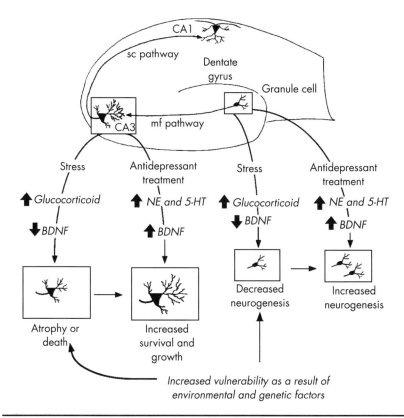

Figure 6–2. *Schematic diagram depicting the atrophy and loss of hippocampal neurons that occur in response to stress. Exposure to stress or to high levels of glucocorticoids has at least two negative effects on hippocampal neurons. First, chronic stress or glucocorticoid treatment leads to atrophy and death of CA3 pyramidal neurons. This effect is thought to result from reduced energy capacity, increased excitotoxicity, and decreased expression of brain-derived neurotrophic factor (BDNF). Second, short-term stress or glucocorticoid exposure decreases neurogenesis of dentate gyrus granule neurons. The action of antidepressant treatments may be mediated, in part, via blockade or reversal of the atrophy and loss of hippocampal neurons. This could occur through induction of BDNF in response to activation of norepinephrine (NE) and serotonin (5-hydroxytryptamine [5-HT]) receptor–coupled second-messenger systems. This model also provides an explanation for individual vulnerability to stress and depression. This vulnerability could be explained by prior exposure to adverse stimuli (e.g., hypoxia, hypoglycemia, excitotoxins) that alone is not sufficient to result in depression. However, with subsequent exposure to stress or other adverse stimuli, neuronal atrophy may reach a level sufficient to produce some of the behavioral characteristics associated with depression. sc = Schaffer collateral; mf = mossy fiber.*

Characterization of these abnormalities is made more difficult by inter-actions between multiple neurotransmitter systems within a given brain region, whether it is the prefrontal cortex, amygdala, or hippo-campus. Much of this characterization has been accomplished with an-imal models of depression. In general, much consideration has been given to determining the validity of animal models of depression and behavioral antidepressant drug screens (Marek and Seiden 1994; Will-ner 1985), yet relatively little work has been directed at determining the neuroanatomic validity of models of depression and antidepressant drug screens. The forced-swim test, originally developed by (Porsolt et al. 1977), does appear to utilize circuits involving the prefrontal cortex, the amygdala, and the paraventricular nucleus of the hypothalamus. For example, the medial prefrontal cortex, lateral orbital cortex, and cin-gulate cortex are activated by the forced-swim test, as demonstrated by an increase in 2-deoxyglucose uptake and *c-fos*–like immunoreactivity (Duncan et al. 1993). The hypothalamic paraventricular nucleus, which contains the corticotropin-releasing hormone (CRH)–secreting neurons controlling adrenocorticotropic hormone (ACTH) release from the pitu-itary, is also activated by the forced-swim test (Duncan et al. 1993). Clearly, work attempting to relate the neuroanatomic basis of behav-ioral models/ screens to the findings of neuroimaging studies is a high priority. This work can be viewed as a guide map for rational selection of brain regions in which to study the molecular biology and physiolog-ical effects of neurotransmitter receptors and signal transduction path-ways linked both to the effects of stress and the therapeutic effects of known and novel antidepressant treatments.

Early theories stated that depression was associated with deple-tions of catecholamines such as norepinephrine (NE) (Schildkraut 1965) and serotonin (5-hydroxytryptamine [5-HT]) (Meltzer and Lowry 1987). Monoamine depletion studies demonstrate that an intact NE or 5-HT system is required for the maintenance of antidepressant respon-siveness (Delgado et al. 1990, 1994; Miller et al. 1996). Antidepressant blockade of monoamine breakdown or reuptake has also provided sup-port for the hypothesis that depression could result from dysregulation of NE or 5-HT neurotransmission. Additionally, chronic antidepressant treatment produces both downregulation of β-adrenergic receptors (Sulser et al. 1978) and desensitization of presynaptic 5-HT$_{1A}$ autorecep-tors (Blier and de Montigny 1994), effects that have been presumed to play a role in the drugs' mechanism of therapeutic action. Clearly, there is some relevance to the catecholamine-depletion hypothesis, as seroto-nin reuptake blockers mediate their antidepressant effects by enhancing serotonergic transmission. However, reduction of monoamine levels alone cannot account for the etiology of depression. For example, depletion of monoamines in most healthy individuals does not induce a depressive condition, and there is no convincing evidence for reduced levels of monoamines in depressed patients. In addition, genetic analysis has failed to demonstrate linkage of depressive symptoms with genes that control monoamine systems, including those for synthetic enzymes, reuptake sites, and receptors.

Alternatively, there is evidence to suggest that other neurotransmitter or regulatory systems and their signal transduction pathways contribute to affective illness. Stress, which can precipitate or worsen depression, has been used as a model for preclinical studies, and progress has been made in understanding the influence of stress on hippocampal neurons. Moreover, these findings are consistent with clinical imaging reports and could help explain the hippocampal atrophy observed in depressed patients. Additional work is needed to further characterize the actions of stress on the hippocampus and to understand how these effects are related to depression. Nonetheless, these studies provide a model for the type of approach that will eventually lead to characterization of the molecular and cellular determinants of stress and depression in hippocampal neurons, as well as other brain regions.

Cellular Actions of Stress on Hippocampal Neurons

Stress is reported to exert different effects on different populations of hippocampal neurons, most notably the CA3 pyramidal and dentate gyrus granule neurons. Of these two, the CA3 pyramidal neurons are more vulnerable to the damaging effects of stress and high levels of glucocorticoids (for reviews, see McEwen 1999; Sapolsky 1996). The influence of stress and glucocorticoids on these neurons can be divided into three different, but related, effects: 1) both chronic exposure to stress and administration of high levels of glucocorticoids cause atrophy of CA3 pyramidal neurons (i.e., decreased number and length of apical dendrites); 2) severe and prolonged stress can cause death of CA3 pyramidal neurons; and 3) low levels of stress or glucocorticoid treatment can result in a state of neuroendangerment wherein the CA3 neurons are more vulnerable to other types of insult (i.e., hypoxia, hypoglycemia, excitotoxins).

Neuroendangerment or low levels of neuronal atrophy or damage could explain why stress induces depression in some individuals but not others. Exposure to stress or other damaging stimuli could produce a state of neuroendangerment or vulnerability, whereupon exposure to subsequent stress leads to further cell atrophy or damage that is sufficient to produce the behavioral characteristics of depression. Alternatively, genetic traits could produce a state of enhanced vulnerability of these neurons so that a first exposure to stress could be sufficient to result in cellular and behavioral abnormalities.

Progenitor cells capable of giving rise to new granule cell neurons are present in the adult hippocampus. These cells been observed in adult brains of several different species, including most recently human hippocampus (Gould et al. 1997, 1998; see Greenough et al. 1999). Progenitor cells in the subgranular zone proliferate and migrate into the granule cell layer and hilus of adult animals. The rate of neurogenesis and the survival of newborn cells are both reported to be decreased by stress and high levels of glucocorticoids (Gould et al. 1997, 1998). In addition, exposure to stress or to high levels of glucocorticoids is reported to decrease neurogenesis.

Atrophy and death of CA3 pyramidal neurons and decreased neurogenesis of granule neurons could lead to a reduction in the size of the hippocampus, consistent with the reduction in hippocampal volume reported in depressed patients. Future studies are required to characterize the morphology and number of hippocampal neurons in depressed patients to test this hypothesis.

Signal Pathways

Stress and glucocorticoids are known to influence a number of signaling systems that contribute to the atrophy and death of CA3 neurons and the reduction of granule cell neurogenesis in the hippocampus (see Duman et al. 1997; McEwen 1999; Sapolsky 1996). Work in this area has focused on three effects: 1) glucocorticoid-induced reduction in glucose utilization, 2) increased glutamate excitotoxicity, and 3) decreased expression of brain-derived neurotrophic factor (BDNF).

Regulation of Glucose Uptake

Adrenal glucocorticoids are known to block glucose uptake in primary neuronal cultures, as well as in fat cells (Horner et al. 1990). The mechanisms underlying this effect have been characterized in fat cells. These studies demonstrate that glucocorticoid exposure induces a translocation of the glucose transporter from the cell membrane to intracellular compartments and decreases the expression of the glucose transporter (Sapolsky 1996). A reduction in glucose uptake would decrease the energy capacity of cells, which could make it more difficult to respond to energy-demanding stimuli (e.g., hypoxia, excitotoxins) and result in a state of neuroendangerment. More long-term and severe reductions in energy capacity, coupled with overactivation of neurons, could result in death of neurons. Decreased glucose uptake has been suggested to contribute to the actions of stress on CA3 neurons, but could also influence the neurogenesis of granule cells.

Regulation of Glutamate Excitotoxicity

The damaging effects of stress on hippocampal neurons are also known to involve the major excitatory amino acid neurotransmitter in the brain, glutamate (Figure 6–3) (McEwen 1999; Sapolsky 1996). Stress is reported to increase the levels of extracellular glutamate in the hippocampus, as measured by microdialysis. Activation of both NMDA and non-NMDA subtypes of glutamate ionotropic receptors increases intracellular calcium. Sustained activation or hyperactivation of these receptors and the resulting elevation of intracellular calcium are known to mediate the excitotoxic effects of aberrant stimuli, including recurrent seizures and ischemia. This excitotoxicity is mediated by activation of multiple intracellular enzymes, many of which can adversely influence cell function and survival. A role for glutamate in the actions of stress on hippocampal neurons is supported by studies demonstrating that pharmacological blockade of glutamate release (i.e., via administration of phenytoin) or of NMDA receptors attenuates atrophy of CA3 neurons and blocks the reduction in neurogenesis in response to stress (McEwen 1999). Glucocorticoids may contribute to the actions of stress on glutamate neurotransmission by regulating the number of pre- and postsynaptic receptors.

Regulation of Neurotrophic Factors

A role for neurotrophic factors in the actions of stress is supported by reports that stress induces a dramatic downregulation of BDNF in the major subfields of the hippocampus (see Figures 6–2 and 6–3) (Duman et al. 1997; Smith et al. 1995). Expression of BDNF is downregulated in response to several different stress paradigms, including immobilization stress (Nibuya et al. 1995; Smith et al. 1995), unpredictable stress (Nibuya et al. 1999), and footshock stress (A. Rasmussen and R. S. Duman, unpublished observation, February 1999). Decreased expression of BDNF could contribute to atrophy and decreased function of hippocampal neurons. However, one study has reported that chronic restraint stress, which induces atrophy of CA3 neurons, does not decrease the expression of BDNF (Kuroda and McEwen 1998). This suggests that loss of BDNF does not contribute to CA3 atrophy, although it is possible that levels of BDNF mRNA or protein are altered at times not examined by

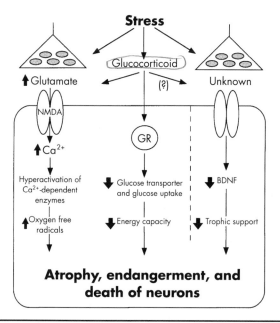

Figure 6–3.   *Schematic diagram depicting the intracellular pathways that contribute to the actions of stress. The actions of stress are thought to involve at least three different systems, all of which could influence the survival and function of hippocampal neurons. First, stress induces high levels of adrenal glucocorticoids, which have widespread effects on neuronal function. One action of glucocorticoids is to decrease levels of the glucose transporter in the membrane. This could result in reduced glucose uptake and decreased energy capacity, an effect that could compromise the ability of neurons to respond to hyperactivation and other stressful cellular conditions. Second, stress is reported to increase the release of glutamate in the hippocampus, which could result in sustained activation of N-methyl-D-aspartate (NMDA) receptors and elevation of intracellular calcium (Ca^{2+}). Hyperactivation of Ca^{2+}-dependent enzymes and generation of oxygen free radicals are known to contribute to the damaging effects of excitotoxins and could play a role in the actions of stress. Glucocorticoids could also directly regulate the release of glutamate and the expression of NMDA receptors. Finally, stress decreases the expression of brain-derived neurotrophic factor (BDNF) in the major subfields of the hippocampus, and this could result in reduced trophic support for CA3 pyramidal and dentate gyrus granule neurons. Although the mechanisms underlying the downregulation of BDNF have not been completely characterized, they could involve 5-HT$_{2A}$ receptors (see text). It is surprising that BDNF is decreased when glutamate is increased, because activation of this neurotransmitter is typically associated with upregulation of BDNF. A possible explanation for this discrepancy is that these two events occur in different populations of cells (indicated by **dashed line**). 5-HT = 5-hydroxytryptamine (serotonin); GR = glucocorticoid receptor.*

Kuroda and McEwen. Additional studies using BDNF knockout mice or reagents that block BDNF function will be required to determine the role of this neurotrophic factor in CA3 atrophy as well as granule cell neurogenesis.

BDNF and other members of the nerve growth factor family have been shown to be critical to the survival and function of neurons in the adult brain, as well as to differentiation of neurons during development (Thoenen 1995). The actions of BDNF are mediated by the tyrosine kinase B (TrkB) receptor, which contains an intracellular tryosine kinase domain that is activated upon binding of BDNF (Figure 6–4). This leads to regulation of coupling proteins and activation of the mitogen-activated protein kinase (MAPK) pathway. This type of intracellular pathway is different from second-messenger pathways that mediate the actions of G protein–coupled receptors.

The mechanisms underlying the downregulation of BDNF have not been well characterized. Glucocorticoid treatment produces a small downregulation of BDNF only in the dentate gyrus, and the actions of stress are not blocked by adrenalectomy. These findings suggest that other factors mediate the effects of stress. Expression of BDNF is known to be dependent on the activity of neuronal systems and is upregulated by activation of both NMDA and non-NMDA glutamate receptors (Metsis et al. 1993). In this regard, evidence demonstrating that stress increases glutamate neurotransmission appears to be contradictory with induction of BDNF expression by glutamate. However, it is possible that release of glutamate occurs in different populations of neurons from those where expression of BDNF is decreased. For example, stress may increase glutamate activation of GABAergic interneurons in the hippocampus that are known to reduce the activity of hippocampal excitatory neurons (see Vaidya et al. 1997). Alternatively, stress may stimulate the release of other regulatory factors that inhibit the expression of BDNF and override the glutamatergic systems that have been activated.

Regulation of Neurogenesis

Neurogenesis of hippocampal progenitor cells is regulated by glucocorticoids and BDNF. Stress or high levels of glucocorticoids decrease neurogenesis (Gould et al. 1997, 1998), although the mechanisms underlying this effect have not been determined. Progenitor cells do not express glucocorticoid receptors, indicating that the inhibitory effects of glucocorticoids are mediated by factors released from other cells. Incubation with BDNF is reported to increase neurogenesis of cultured progenitor cells, raising the possibility that downregulation of BDNF could

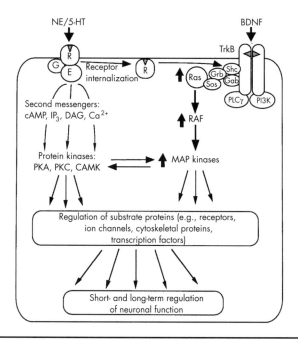

Figure 6–4. *Model of receptor-coupled intracellular signal transduction cascades. Different types of signaling pathways mediate the actions of monoamine (NE/5-HT) G protein–coupled receptors and BDNF–TrkB receptors. G protein receptors couple to second messenger–dependent pathways (i.e., cAMP, IP$_3$, DAG, Ca^{2+}) and their respective protein kinases (PKA, PKC, and CAMK). TrkB receptors have intrinsic tyrosine kinase activity that is stimulated upon binding of BDNF. This results in the regulation of different signal transduction pathways, including PLCγ, PI3K, and the MAPK pathway, via tyrosine phosphorylation of adaptor and effector proteins. Phosphorylation of the adaptor proteins, Shc, Gab, and Grb, results in recruitment of Sos, a guanine nucleotide exchange factor that stimulates the small guanosine 5′-triphosphate (GTP)–binding protein Ras. This leads to activation of Raf and the MAP kinases (also referred to as extracellular signal–regulated protein kinase 1 and 2 [ERK1 and ERK2]). There is also evidence for cross-talk between the second messenger–dependent protein kinases and the MAP kinases. In addition, internalization of monoamine receptors can result in the recruitment of a soluble tyrosine kinase (Src) that phosphorylates the adaptor proteins and can thereby activate the MAPK pathway. NE = norepinephrine; 5-HT = 5-hydroxytryptamine (serotonin); R = receptor; G = G protein; E = effector; BDNF = brain-derived neurotrophic factor; TrkB = tyrosine kinase B; PLCα = phospholipase C–α; PI3K = phosphatidylinositol 3-kinase; cAMP = cyclic adenosine 3′,5′-monophosphate; IP$_3$ = inositol 1,4,5-triphosphate; DAG = diacylglycerol; Ca^{2+} = calcium; PKA = protein kinase A; PKC = protein kinase C; CAMK = Ca^{2+}/calmodulin–dependent protein kinase; MAPK = mitogen-activated protein kinase.*

contribute to the stress-induced decrease of neurogenesis (Palmer et al. 1997). Alternatively, other trophic factor systems, such as transforming growth factor alpha (TGFα), may play a role in regulation of neurogenesis.

Although the studies described reveal significant progress, this work represents only the initial characterization of the signal transduction pathways that are involved in the actions of stress and depression. Future studies will be required to further characterize the complex intracellular pathways, and interactions of these systems, that underlie the actions of stress and the etiology of depression.

Psychopharmacology

The acute actions of most typical antidepressant drugs are mediated by blockade of the reuptake or breakdown of NE and/or 5-HT. Development of selective inhibitors of 5-HT and NE reuptake/transporter sites has resulted in a new generation of antidepressants that have fewer side effects. However, the therapeutic action of antidepressants is dependent on long-term administration, suggesting that adaptations to the upregulation of monoamines are required for therapeutic responses to these agents. Based on this hypothesis, characterization of the neural adaptations at the cellular and molecular levels, as well as the interpretation of these adaptations in the context of stress, has been a major focus of antidepressant research.

Morphology and Number of Hippocampal Neurons

A few studies have been conducted to examine the ability of antidepressants to influence the cellular processes regulated by stress, including CA3 pyramidal cell atrophy and granule cell neurogenesis. The results demonstrate that antidepressant treatment can block the effect of stress or can alone exert positive actions, although additional characterization of these findings is required. Very little is known about the effects of antidepressants on the morphology and survival of neurons in other brain regions, such as the prefrontal cortex, where the size and number of neurons are reported to be reduced in postmortem brains of depressed patients.

CA3 Pyramidal Neurons

Atrophy of CA3 pyramidal neurons in rats is reported to be blocked by chronic administration of the putative antidepressant tianeptine

(Watanabe et al. 1992). Tianeptine is an atypical agent that enhances the reuptake of 5-HT, in contrast to the blocking action of typical antidepressant agents such as fluoxetine. Preliminary studies suggest that other classes of antidepressants, including 5-HT selective reuptake inhibitors, do not influence CA3 pyramidal cell atrophy (see McEwen 1999). Chronic administration of tianeptine or fluoxetine does not appear to influence the dendritic arborization of CA3 neurons. These findings are difficult to interpret, but raise the possibility that increased release of 5-HT in response to stress, but not in response to fluoxetine, contributes to atrophy of CA3 neurons. Further analysis of typical antidepressants, including different dosage and time regimens, should be conducted to examine this hypothesis and to determine whether blockade of CA3 atrophy is specific to tianeptine. Alternatively, antidepressant treatment may have more subtle effects on neuronal morphology, such as regulation of the density of spines on CA3 dendrites, a possibility that requires future testing.

Hippocampal Granule Cells

Studies in rodents also demonstrate that antidepressants increase neurogenesis and sprouting of dentate gyrus granule cells in the hippocampus of rats. Chronic, but not acute, administration of different classes of antidepressants, including 5-HT and NE selective reuptake inhibitors and a monoamine oxidase inhibitor, and chronic administration of electroconvulsive seizures (ECS) significantly increase the number of newborn cells in the dentate gyrus (Duman et al. 1999; Malberg et al. 2000). This effect has been replicated by other investigators (Jacobs et al. 2000; Madsen et al. 2000; Manev et al. 2001). One of those investigators also found that administration of a 5-HT$_{1A}$ receptor agonist increased granule cell neurogenesis (Jacobs et al. 2000). Additional studies are required to further characterize the influence of antidepressants on neurogenesis, to determine the signal transduction pathways that underlie this effect, and to examine the functional consequences of increased cell birth.

Chronic ECS is also reported to increase the sprouting of dentate gyrus granule cells in rats (Vaidya et al. 1999). In contrast to kindling and excitotoxin paradigms, wherein the induction of sprouting is accompanied by cell death, there is no evidence that chronic ECS administration results in the death or damage of neurons. This suggests that granule sprouting is not a compensatory response to cell loss, but rather is induced by factors released during ECS. In this regard, ECS induction of granule cell sprouting is partially blocked in BDNF-heterozygous knockout mice, suggesting that this neurotrophic factor is necessary for sprouting. It is likely that other factors, such as glutamate, also play a significant role in granule cell sprouting. However, chronic administration of chemical antidepressants does not significantly influence sprouting, indicating that this effect is selective for ECS.

Signal Transduction Pathways Involved in Antidepressant Action

The cellular actions of NE and 5-HT are mediated by multiple receptor subtypes, largely of the G protein–coupled receptor family, and their corresponding second-messenger signal transduction pathways. These pathways include the cAMP, phosphatidylinositol, and Ca^{2+} second-messenger cascades (see Figure 6–4) (Duman et al. 1997; Manji et al. 1995). Although there are reports of antidepressant regulation of several of these systems, evidence supports a significant role for the cAMP pathway in the action of antidepressant treatment. In addition, the cAMP response element binding protein (CREB), a transcription factor that is regulated by the cAMP system, can be activated by other second-messenger systems and could thereby act as a common downstream target of monoamines and antidepressant treatments.

Antidepressant Upregulation of the cAMP Cascade

The cAMP cascade is upregulated at several different levels by chronic antidepressant treatment (Figure 6–5). This includes increased coupling of the stimulatory G protein (G_s) to adenylyl cyclase, resulting in upregulation of cAMP formation (Ozawa and Rasenick 1991). Levels of cAMP-dependent protein kinase (PKA) are also upregulated in response to chronic, but not acute, antidepressant treatment (Nestler et al. 1989; Perez et al. 1989). Antidepressant treatment is also reported to increase the level of PKA in crude nuclear fractions of the frontal cortex, suggesting that gene transcription factors are regulated under these conditions. This possibility is supported by the finding that antidepressant treatment increases the expression and function of the transcription factor CREB (Nibuya et al. 1996). A potential role for CREB in the pathophysiology, as well as treatment, of depression is supported by a recent report that levels of this transcription factor are reduced in postmortem brains of depressed patients (Dowlatshahi et al. 1998). Moreover, this effect appears to be reversed in patients receiving antidepressant treatment at the time of death.

Upregulation of the cAMP pathway appears to be contradictory to the well-established action of antidepressants to downregulate the

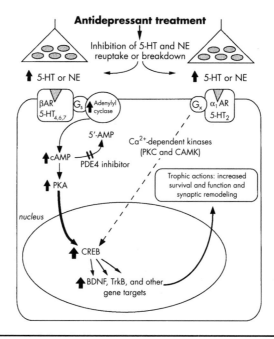

Figure 6–5.   *Schematic diagram depicting the intracellular pathways that contribute to the actions of antidepressant treatment. Antidepressants increase synaptic levels of norepinephrine (NE) and serotonin (5-HT) by blocking the reuptake or breakdown of these monoamines. This leads to regulation of receptor-coupled signal transduction pathways. One pathway that is regulated by antidepressant treatment is the cAMP signal transduction cascade. Antidepressant treatment increases the coupling of the stimulatory G protein (G_s) with adenylyl cyclase, increases particulate levels of protein kinase A (PKA), and increases expression of CREB. This model implies that activation of the cAMP pathway could result in antidepressant efficacy. This hypothesis is supported by basic research and clinical trials demonstrating that inhibitors of PDE4, the enzyme that breaks down cAMP, have antidepressant efficacy. Induction of CREB by antidepressant treatment indicates that target genes are also regulated by antidepressant treatment. BDNF and TrkB are upregulated by antidepressant treatment, and these effects are thought to occur via the cAMP-CREB cascade. CREB could serve as a common NE and 5-HT postreceptor target because it can also be activated by Ca^{2+}-dependent protein kinases. These kinases could be regulated by α_1-adrenergic (α_1AR) and $5\text{-}HT_{2A}$ receptors, as well as by activation of glutamate receptors (not shown). 5-HT = 5-hydroxytryptamine (serotonin); AR = adrenergic; G_x = G protein x; 5'-AMP = 5'-adenosine monophosphate; Ca^{2+} = calcium; PKC = protein kinase C; CAMK = Ca^{2+}/ calmodulin-dependent protein kinase; cAMP = cyclic adenosine 3',5'-monophosphate; PDE4 = phosphodiesterase 4; CREB = cAMP response element binding; BDNF = brain-derived neurotrophic factor; TrkB = tyrosine kinase B.*

number of β-adrenergic receptors (βARs) and their coupling to cAMP production. However, the possibility that downregulation or antagonism of βAR alone could account for the therapeutic action of antidepressant treatment has largely been discounted (for discussion, see Duman et al. 1997, 1999). Moreover, the reduction in βAR number implies that there is sustained stimulation of the cAMP pathway, and upregulation of the intracellular cascade indicates that the remaining receptors are sufficient to regulate the system.

CREB is a Common Downstream Target of Several Signal Transduction Pathways

CREB can be regulated by NE and 5-HT receptors that are directly coupled to the cAMP cascade, including the $5\text{-HT}_{4,6,7}$ receptor subtypes, as well as the $\beta_1 AR$ and $\beta_2 AR$ subtypes (see Figure 6–5). In addition to its regulation by the cAMP second-messenger cascade, CREB is regulated by other NE and 5-HT receptor–coupled second-messenger pathways. In this way, CREB could serve as a common target of monoamine-receptor signaling systems and antidepressants. The transcriptional activity of CREB is stimulated by phosphorylation at Ser^{133}, which is mediated by PKA, as well as other second messenger–dependent protein kinases. Most notable are the Ca^{2+}-dependent protein kinases, including $Ca^{2+}/$ calmodulin-dependent protein kinase (CAMK) and protein kinase C (PKC) (see Figure 6–5). In fact, activation of CAMK in response to glutamatergic neurotransmission and neuronal depolarization exerts a potent stimulatory effect on CREB. PKC and CAMK are also activated by NE and 5-HT receptors that are coupled to the phosphatidylinositol system, including αAR_1 and 5-HT_2 receptor subtypes.

Role of Brain-Derived Neurotrophic Factor in Antidepressant Action

Activation of the cAMP-CREB cascade indicates that regulation of specific genes also plays a role in the action of antidepressant treatment. One target that is regulated by antidepressant treatment is BDNF. Chronic administration of different classes of antidepressants, including NE and 5-HT selective reuptake inhibitors, increases the expression of BDNF in limbic brain regions (Nibuya et al. 1995, 1996). Importantly, BDNF expression is increased in the subfields of the hippocampus (CA3 pyramidal and dentate gyrus granule cell layers), where stress is reported to induce atrophy and loss of cells. These studies also demonstrate that antidepressant treatment blocks the stress-induced downregulation of BDNF in these hippocampal subfields. Finally, expression of the BDNF receptor TrkB is also upregulated by antidepressant treatment (Nibuya et al. 1995, 1996). Although the exact molecular mechanisms underlying the induction of BDNF by antidepressant treatment have not been identified, recent studies have characterized a cAMP response element in the promoter region of the BDNF gene that could account for this effect (Shieh et al. 1998; Tao et al. 1998).

A role for BDNF in the action of antidepressant treatment is also supported by functional studies. First, infusion of BDNF into the midbrain is reported to have antidepressant effects in two behavioral models of depression, the forced swim and the learned helplessness paradigms (Siuciak et al. 1997). Second, BDNF has potent neurotrophic effects on both NE and 5-HT neurons, increasing the survival and function of these neurons (see Duman et al. 1997, 1999). These findings suggest that BDNF could act on both presynaptic and postsynaptic sites of monoamine neurotransmission.

These studies provide support for the hypothesis that antidepressants may act, in part, via a neurotrophic-like mechanism. However, additional studies are needed to further test this hypothesis. In addition, it is likely that other target genes are regulated by CREB and antidepressant treatment, and future studies will be needed to further characterize the program of genes regulated by these psychotropic drugs.

Novel Antidepressant Agents

The discovery that antidepressant treatment results in upregulation, not downregulation, of the cAMP-CREB cascade and induction of the BDNF-MAPK system provides novel targets for drug development and testing. For example, agents that activate or upregulate the cAMP pathway would be predicted to have antidepressant efficacy. This hypothesis has already been tested with the development of inhibitors of cAMP phosphodiesterase 4 (PDE4), the enzymes that block the breakdown of cAMP. PDE inhibitors, such as rolipram, are reported to have antidepressant efficacy in behavioral models and in clinical trials (Duman et al. 1997, 1999). Although the use of rolipram has been limited by its side effects, these findings support the notion that upregulation of the cAMP cascade can produce an antidepressant response. In addition, identification of multiple genes and splice variants of PDE4 raises the possibility that other drugs that specifically target one of these isozymes could be an effective antidepressant without the side effects (Takahashi et al. 1999).

Another possibility would be to target receptors that are directly coupled to the cAMP pathway. As mentioned above, several 5-HT receptors are positively coupled to the cAMP system, including the $5\text{-}HT_4$, $5\text{-}HT_6$, and $5\text{-}HT_7$ subtypes. All three of these receptors are expressed in limbic brain regions, although the $5\text{-}HT_4$ receptor is also expressed in peripheral tissues (gut), and drugs acting on this subtype could have side effects. One additional concern with direct-acting receptor agonists is that their effectiveness could be attenuated by downregulation of receptor binding sites. However, the usefulness of this approach can only be determined by direct testing after such agents become available.

Assuming that the BDNF-MAPK pathway contributes to the action of antidepressants, yet another possibility is to target components of this system. Although very few known activators of this system are available, inhibitors of MAPK exist that could be used to examine the role of this pathway in behavioral and neurochemical responses to antidepressants. Another way to enhance the function of the BDNF-MAPK pathway is to block the enzymes that inactivate MAP kinases (i.e., phosphatases). However, these phosphatases, as well as the MAP kinases, are widely distributed, and additional studies will be needed to determine if they are valid targets for development of antidepressant agents.

These are just a few of the many possible novel sites that could be targeted for drug development. Identification of additional targets will depend on further characterization of the actions of antidepressant treatment on receptor-coupled intracellular signal transduction systems and the genes that are regulated by these pathways.

Conclusions

The progress outlined in this review provides new approaches and hypotheses for the field of depression. Brain imaging and postmortem studies have identified several limbic brain structures that appear to be involved in depression, but additional work is needed to further characterize the functional role and interactions of these regions in mood disorders. This work has also resulted in the astonishing discovery that neurochemical imbalances in depressed patients are accompanied by structural alterations in limbic brain regions, including the prefrontal cortex and hippocampus. Importantly, preclinical and clinical studies indicate that structural alterations in the hippocampus, and possibly other brain regions, are reversible. Further studies at the molecular and cellular levels are being conducted to characterize the receptor-coupled intracellular signaling pathways that underlie the structural alterations, as well as the actions of antidepressant treatment. These studies hold the promise of identifying novel targets that could prove more effective and faster acting for the treatment of depression. Continued multidisciplinary studies using cutting-edge neurobiological approaches will provide a more complete understanding of the pathophysiology and treatment of depression.

References

Abercrombie HC, Schaefer SM, Larson CL, et al: Metabolic rate in the right amygdala predicts negative affect in depressed patients. Neuroreport 9: 3301–3307, 1998

American Psychiatric Association: Diagnostic and Statistical Manual of Mental Disorders, 4th Edition. Washington, DC, American Psychiatric Association, 1994

American Psychiatric Association: Diagnostic and Statistical Manual of Mental Disorders, 4th Edition, Text Revision. Washington, DC, American Psychiatric Association, 2000

Baxter LR Jr, Phelps ME, Mazziotta JC, et al: Cerebral metabolic rates for glucose in mood disorders: studies with positron emission tomography and fluorodeoxyglucose F 18. Arch Gen Psychiatry 42:441–447, 1985

Baxter LR Jr, Schwartz JM, Phelps ME, et al: Reduction of prefrontal cortex glucose metabolism common to three types of depression. Arch Gen Psychiatry 46:243–250, 1989

Bench CJ, Friston KJ, Brown RG, et al: The anatomy of melancholia-focal abnormalities of cerebral blood flow in major depression. Psychiatr Med 22:607–615, 1992

Biver F, Friston KJ, Brown RG, et al: Frontal and parietal metabolic disturbances in unipolar depression. Biol Psychiatry 36:381–388, 1994

Blier P, de Montigny C: Current advances and trends in the treatment of depression. Trends Pharmacol Sci 15:220–226, 1994

Bonne O, Krausz Y, Shapira B, et al: Increased cerebral blood flow in depressed patients responding to electroconvulsive therapy. J Nucl Med 37:1075–1080, 1996

Bremner JD, Randall P, Scott TM, et al: MRI-based measurement of hippocampal volume in patients with combat-related posttraumatic stress disorder. Am J Psychiatry 152:973–981, 1995

Bremner JD, Innis RB, Salomon RM, et al: Positron emission tomography measurement of cerebral metabolic correlates of tryptophan depletion-induced depressive relapse. Arch Gen Psychiatry 54:364–374, 1997

Bremner JD, Narayan M, Anderson ER, et al: Hippocampal volume reduction in major depression. Am J Psychiatry 157:115–118, 2000

Buchsbaum MS, Wu J, DeLisi LE, et al: Frontal cortex and basal ganglia metabolic rates assessed by positron emission tomography with [18F]2-deoxyglucose in affective illness. J Affect Disord 10:137–152, 1986

Coffey CE, Wilkinson WE, Weiner RD, et al: Quantitative cerebral anatomy in depression. A controlled magnetic resonance imaging study. Arch Gen Psychiatry 50:7–16, 1993

Cummings JL: The neuroanatomy of depression. J Clin Psychiatry 54 (suppl): 14–20, 1993

Delgado PL, Charney DS, Price LH, et al: Serotonin function and the mechanism of antidepressant action: reversal of antidepressant-induced remission by rapid depletion of plasma tryptophan. Arch Gen Psychiatry 47:411–418, 1990

Delgado PL, Price LH, Miller HL, et al: Serotonin and the neurobiology of depression: effects of tryptophan depletion in drug-free depressed patients. Arch Gen Psychiatry 51:865–874, 1994

Dowlatshahi D, MacQueen GM, Wang JF, et al: Increased temporal cortex CREB concentrations and antidepressant treatment in major depression. Lancet 352:1754–1755,1998

Drevets WC: Functional neuroimaging studies of major depression: the anatomy of melancholia. Annu Rev Med 49:341–361, 1998

Drevets WC, Videen TO, Price JL, et al: A functional anatomical study of unipolar depression. J Neurosci 12:3628–3641, 1992

Drevets WC, Price JL, Simpson JR Jr, et al: Subgenual prefrontal cortex abnormalities in mood disorders. Nature 386:824–827, 1997

Duman RS, Heninger GR, Nestler EJ: A molecular and cellular theory of depression. Arch Gen Psychiatry 54:597–606, 1997

Duman RS, Malberg J, Thome J: Neural plasticity to stress and antidepressant treatment. Biol Psychiatry 46:1181–1191, 1999

Duncan GE, Johnson KB, Breese GR: Topographic patterns of brain activity in response to swim stress: assessment by 2-deoxyglucose uptake and expression of fos-like immunoreactivity. J Neurosci 13:3932–3943, 1993

Elkis H, Friedman L, Wise A, et al: Meta-analyses of studies of ventricular enlargement and cortical sulcal prominence in mood disorders: comparisons with controls or patients with schizophrenia. Arch Gen Psychiatry 52:735–746,1995

Goodwin FK, Jamison KR: Manic-Depressive Illness. New York, Oxford University Press, 1990

Gould E, McEwen BS, Tanapat P, et al: Neurogenesis in the dentate gyrus of the adult tree shrew is regulated by psychosocial stress and NMDA receptor activation. J Neurosci 17:2492–2498, 1997

Gould E, Tanapat P, McEwen BS, et al: Proliferation of granule cell precursors in the dentate gyrus of adult monkeys is diminished by stress. Proc Natl Acad Sci U S A 95:3168–3171, 1998

Greenough WT, Cohen NJ, Juraska JM: New neurons in old brains: learning to survive? Nat Neurosci 2:203–205, 1999

Gurvits TV, Shenton ME, Hokama H, et al: Magnetic resonance imaging study of the hippocampal volume in chronic, combat-related posttraumatic stress disorder. Biol Psychiatry 40:1091–1099, 1996

Ho AP, Gillin JC, Buchsbaum MS, et al: Brain glucose metabolism during non-rapid eye movement sleep in major depression. A positron emission tomography study. Arch Gen Psychiatry 53:645–652, 1996

Horner H, Packan D, Sapolsky R: Glucocorticoids inhibit glucose transport in cultured hippocampal neurons and glia. Neuroendocrinology 52:57–62, 1990

Husain MM, McDonald WM, Doraiswamy PM, et al: A magnetic resonance imaging study of putamen nuclei in major depression. Psychiatry Res 40:95–99, 1991

Jacobs BL, Praag H, Gage FH: Adult brain neurogenesis and psychiatry: a novel theory of depression. Mol Psychiatry 5:262–269, 2000

Judd LL: The clinical course of major depressive disorders. Arch Gen Psychiatry 54:989–992, 1997

Krishnan KR, Doraiswamy PM, Lurie SN, et al: Pituitary size in depression. J Clin Endocrinol Metab 72:256–259, 1991

Krishnan KR, McDonald WM, Escalona PR, et al: Magnetic resonance imaging of the caudate nuclei in depression. Preliminary observations. Arch Gen Psychiatry 49:553–557, 1992

Kuroda Y, McEwen BS: Effect of chronic restraint stress and tianeptine on growth factors, growth-associated protein-43 and microtubule-associated protein 2 mRNA expression in the rat hippocampus. Brain Res Mol Brain Res 59:35–39, 1998

Madsen TM, Treschow A, Bengzon J, et al: Increased neurogenesis in a model of electroconvulsive therapy. Biol Psychiatry 47:1043–1049, 2000

Malberg JE, Eisch AJ, Nestler EJ, et al: Chronic antidepressant treatment increases neurogenesis in adult rat hippocampus. J Neurosci 20:9104–9110, 2000

Manev H, Uz T, Smalheiser NR, et al: Antidepressants alter cell proliferation in the adult brain in vivo and in neural cultures in vitro. Eur J Pharmacol 411:67–70, 2001

Manji HK, Potter WC, Lenox RH: Signal transduction pathways. Arch Gen Psychiatry 52:531–543, 1995

Marek GJ, Seiden LS: Antidepressant drug screens and the serotonergic system, in Strategies for Studying Brain Disorders, Vol 1: Affective Disorders and Drug Abuse. Edited by Palomo T, Archer T, Hodson K. London, Farrand Press, 1994, pp 23–40

Mayberg HS: Limbic-cortical dysregulation: a proposed model of depression. J Neuropsychiatry Clin Neurosci 9:471–481, 1997

Mayberg HS, Brannan SK, Mahurin RK, et al: Cingulate function in depression: a potential predictor of treatment response. Neuroreport 8:1057–1061, 1997

McEwen BS: Stress and hippocampal plasticity. Annu Rev Neurosci 22:105–122, 1999

Meltzer HY, Lowry MT: The serotonin hypothesis of depression, in Psychopharmacology: The Third Generation of Progress. Edited by Meltzer HY. New York, Raven, 1987, pp 513–526

Metsis M, Timmusk T, Arenas E, et al: Differential usage of multiple brain-derived neurotrophic factor promoters in the rat brain following neuronal activation. Proc Natl Acad Sci U S A 90:8802–8806, 1993

Miller HL, Delgado PL, Salomon RM, et al: The behavioral effects of catecholamine depletion on antidepressant induced remission of depression: implications for monoamine hypothesis of antidepressant action. Arch Gen Psychiatry 53:117–128, 1996

Nelson JC, Davis JM: DST studies in psychotic depression: a meta-analysis. Am J Psychiatry 154:1497–1503, 1997

Nemeroff CB, Krishnan KR, Reed D, et al: Adrenal gland enlargement in major depression: a computed tomographic study. Arch Gen Psychiatry 49:384–387, 1992

Nestler EJ, Terwilliger RZ, Duman RS: Chronic antidepressant administration alters the subcellular distribution of cyclic AMP-dependent protein kinase in rat frontal cortex. J Neurochem 53:1644–1647, 1989

Nibuya M, Morinobu S, Duman RS: Regulation of BDNF and TrkB mRNA in rat brain by chronic electroconvulsive seizure and antidepressant drug treatments. J Neurosci 15:7539–7547, 1995

Nibuya M, Nestler EJ, Duman RS: Chronic antidepressant administration increases the expression of cAMP response element binding protein (CREB) in rat hippocampus. J Neurosci 16:2365–2372, 1996

Nibuya M, Takahashi M, Russell DS, et al: Repeated stress increases catalytic TrkB mRNA in rat hippocampus. Neurosci Lett 265:1–4, 1999

Nobler MS, Sackheim HA, Prohovnik I, et al: Regional cerebral blood flow in mood disorders, III: treatment and clinical response. Arch Gen Psychiatry 51:884–897, 1994

Ongur D, Drevets WC, Price JL: Glial reduction in the subgenual prefrontal cortex in mood disorders. Proc Nat Acad Sci U S A 95:13290–13295, 1998

Ozawa H, Rasenick MM: Chronic electroconvulsive treatment augments coupling of the GTP-binding protein Gs to the catalytic moiety of adenylyl cyclase in a manner similar to that seen with chronic antidepressant drugs. J Neurochem 56:330–338, 1991

Palmer TD, Takahashi J, Gage FH: The adult rat hippocampus contains primordial neural stem cells. Mol Cell Neurosci 8:389–404, 1997

Perez J, Tinelli D, Brunello N, et al: cAMP-dependent phosphorylation of soluble and crude microtubule fractions of rat cerebral cortex after prolonged desmethylimipramine treatment. Eur J Pharmacol 172:305–316, 1989

Porsolt RD, Le Pichon M, Jalfre M: Depression: a new animal model sensitive to antidepressant treatments. Nature 266:730–732, 1977

Rajkowska G, Miguel-Hidalgo JJ, Wei J, et al: Morphometric evidence for neuronal and glial prefrontal cell pathology in major depression. Biol Psychiatry 45:1085–1098, 1999

Raz S, Raz N: Structural brain abnormalities in the major psychoses: a quantitative review of the evidence from computerized imaging. Psychol Bull 108: 93–108, 1990

Sapolsky RM: Stress, glucocorticoids, and damage to the nervous system: the current state of confusion. Stress 1:1–19, 1996

Schildkraut JJ: The catecholamine hypothesis of affective disorders: a review of supporting evidence. Am J Psychiatry 122:509–522, 1965

Sheline YI, Wang PW, Gado MH, et al: Hippocampal atrophy in recurrent major depression. Proc Natl Acad Sci U S A 93:3909–3913, 1996

Shieh PB, Hu S-C, Bobb K, et al: Identification of a signaling pathway involved in calcium regulation of BDNF expression. Neuron 20:727–740, 1998

Siuciak JA, Lewis DR, Wiegand SJ, et al: Antidepressant-like effect of brain-derived neurotrophic factor (BDNF). Pharmacol Biochem Behav 56:131–137, 1997

Smith MA, Makino S, Kvetnansky R, et al: Stress and glucocorticoids affect the expression of brain-derived neurotrophic factor and neurotrophin-3 mRNAs in the hippocampus. J Neurosci 15:1768–1777, 1995

Starkman MN, Gebarski SS, Berent S, et al: Hippocampal formation volume, memory dysfunction, and cortisol levels in patients with Cushing's syndrome. Biol Psychiatry 32:756–765, 1992

Sulser F, Vetulani JA, Mobley P: Mode of action of antidepressant drugs. Biochem Pharmacol 27:257–261, 1978

Takahashi M, Terwilliger R, Lane C, et al: Chronic antidepressant administration increases the expression of cAMP phosphodiesterase 4A and 4B isoforms. J Neurosci 19:610–618, 1999

Tao X, Finkbeiner S, Arnold DB, et al: Ca2+ influx regulates BDNF transcription by a CREB family transcription factor-dependent mechanism. Neuron 20: 709–726, 1998

Thoenen H: Neurotrophins and neuronal plasticity. Science 270:593–598, 1995

Vaidya VA, Marek GJ, Aghajanian GA, et al: 5-HT2A receptor-mediated regulation of brain-derived neurotrophic factor mRNA in the hippocampus and the neocortex. J Neurosci 17:2785–2795, 1997

Vaidya VA, Siuciak J, Du F, et al: Mossy fiber sprouting and synaptic reorganization induced by chronic administration of electroconvulsive seizure: role of BDNF. Neuroscience 89:157–166, 1999

Watanabe Y, Gould E, Daniels DC, et al: Tianeptine attenuates stress-induced morphological changes in the hippocampus. Eur J Pharmacol 222:157–162, 1992

Willner P: Depression: A Psychobiological Synthesis. New York, Wiley, 1985

Winokur G: All roads lead to depression: clinically homogeneous, etiologically heterogeneous. J Affect Disord 45:97–108, 1997

Young EA, Haskett RF, Murphy-Weinberg V, et al: Loss of glucocorticoid fast feedback in depression. Arch Gen Psychiatry 48:693–699, 1991

CHAPTER 7

Neural Circuitry and Signaling in Bipolar Disorder

Roberto B. Sassi, M.D.
Jair C. Soares, M.D.

Clinical Presentation

Bipolar affective disorder is a common psychiatric illness with an estimated lifetime prevalence rate of approximately 1.0%–1.5% (Weissman et al. 1988). The prevalence of bipolar disorder is similar among various races and geographic locations, and it affects males and females in equal proportions. Bipolar affective disorder is characterized by recurrent and often disabling episodes of manic, hypomanic, depressive, or mixed symptoms (Paykel 1992). Two main clinical subtypes of bipolar disorders have been described. These two subtypes usually have a distinct course and natural history (Coryell et al. 1995): a bipolar subtype I characterized by the occurrence of at least one manic or mixed episode, and a bipolar subtype II with only hypomanic episodes. Virtually all patients, type I or II, will also present with at least one major depressive episode. A manic episode can be described as a period of abnormally expansive affect, sometimes presenting with irritability, often accompanied by increased energy and self-esteem, restlessness, racing thoughts, pressured speech, reduced need for sleep, impulsive behavior, and, not infrequently, psychotic symptoms. A hypomanic episode could be considered a milder form of mania, although the course of bipolar type II can be as disabling as the course of bipolar type I. An affective episode

This work was partially supported by National Institutes of Health (NIH) Grants MH 01736 and MH 30915, the Stanley Foundation, the National Alliance for Research on Schizophrenia and Depression (NARSAD), and the CAPES Foundation (Fundação Coordenação de Aperfeiçoamento de Pessoal de Nível Superior; Brazil).

that meets criteria for both mania and depression is classified as a mixed episode.

Although an increased understanding of the biological basis of bipolar disorder has emerged in the last decade, its etiology still remains largely unclear. Most studies on bipolar disorders have been conducted with type I patients. There is still controversy about whether the depressive states in bipolar patients share the same biological mechanisms as unipolar depression, or if bipolar depression should be considered a distinct entity. In this chapter we review available findings from neurobiological studies that attempt to elucidate the mechanisms involved in bipolar disorder.

Neural Circuitry

Findings from postmortem and brain-imaging studies converge toward a postulated mood-regulating pathway involving a prefrontal cortex–striatum–pallidum–thalamus–limbic circuit (Drevets et al. 1998; Soares and Mann 1997; Warsh 2000). These brain regions are connected via fast-conductance neurotransmitters (glutamate and γ-aminobutyric acid [GABA]) and are modulated by the action of catecholamines, serotonin (5-hydroxytryptamine [5-HT]), acetylcholine (ACh), neuropeptides, and hormones (Anand and Charney 2000). Mood disorders appear to involve abnormalities in this postulated circuit. Some diseases known to affect the brain regions included in this neuroanatomic model—such as stroke, closed-head injury, and Parkinson's, Huntington's, or Fahr's diseases—are frequently reported to lead to secondary depression or mania (e.g., Mayberg et al. 1992).

Postmortem Structural Findings

Despite their crucial role in addressing relevant questions concerning anatomic and histopathological issues, postmortem studies have been largely neglected in bipolar disorder. Nonetheless, one study (Benes et al. 1998) found reductions in nonpyramidal cells in the hippocampal CA2 region in postmortem brains of both schizophrenic and bipolar subjects, even in those not exposed to neuroleptics. A trend toward lower nonpyramidal density was also detected in the CA3 region only in bipolar subjects in this preliminary study. Another study (Rajkowska et al. 1997) showed a marked decrease in cortical and laminar thickness in the dorsolateral prefrontal cortex in schizophrenic and bipolar subjects. Interestingly, the reduction was produced by a decrease in glial density in layer III of the cortex. The overall neuronal density observed in bipolar patients was similar to that in control subjects (unlike schizophrenic patients). This study provides evidence for differential patterns of cortical pathology in these disorders. More recently, the same investigators found a decrease in both neuronal and glial densities in the dorsolateral prefrontal cortex of major depressive unipolar subjects (Rajkowska et al. 1999). Glial reduction has also been reported in the subgenual part of the prefrontal cortex (Brodmann area 24) of subjects with depressive disorders, both unipolar and bipolar, but only in those with a family history of affective disorders (Ongur et al. 1998). There were no changes in the number or size of neurons in this region in mood disorder subjects. These preliminary findings are in agreement with positron-emission tomography (PET) and magnetic resonance imaging (MRI) studies conducted by the same investigators in bipolar and unipolar depressed subjects (Drevets et al. 1997, 1998). The specific pathological mechanisms that could lead to damage of neural and glial cells in these brain regions in bipolar disorder are still unknown. Also, the possibility that these reductions could represent neurodevelopmental abnormalities still requires investigation.

Brain Imaging Studies

The first studies performed with computed tomography (CT) in bipolar patients pointed to alterations in the cerebellum, basal ganglia, and temporal lobe (Dewan et al. 1988). MRI studies found abnormalities in specific subregions of the frontal lobe: decreased prefrontal cortex in manic subjects (Sax et al. 1999), and decreased gray matter content in the subgenual prefrontal cortex in depressed unipolar and bipolar subjects with a family history of affective disorders (Drevets et al. 1997).

Some controversy surrounds temporal lobe findings in bipolar patients. Some studies have reported increased gray matter volumes (Harvey et al. 1994), others have showed smaller temporal lobe volumes in bipolar patients compared with healthy control subjects (Altshuler et al. 1991), and still others have found no significant differences between bipolar patients and healthy control subjects (Swayze et al. 1992). In regard to studies examining specific regions within the temporal lobe, there is a report of increased amygdala volumes in bipolar patients compared with healthy controls (Strakowski et al. 1999). However, other studies have reported smaller left amygdalar volumes (Pearlson et al. 1997) or no abnormalities in measures of amygdala area in bipolar subjects (Swayze et al. 1992). Structural findings in the hippocampus likewise are conflicting: decreased volume of the right hippocampus (Swayze et al. 1992) in one study, and no significant differences in others (Strakowski et al. 1999). The technical difficulties involved in measuring these small medial temporal lobe structures with MRI probably account for the discrepant findings.

Anatomic abnormalities in the basal ganglia may be more common in unipolar depression than in bipolar disorder. Although some studies found no abnormalities in caudate volumes in bipolar patients (Harvey et al. 1994; Swayze et al. 1992), one study found significantly enlarged caudate volumes (Aylward et al. 1994). There have been reports of smaller caudate (Krishnan et al. 1992) and putamen (Husain et al. 1991) volumes in unipolar depressive disorder patients, although a relatively recent study in unipolar patients did not find abnormalities in gray matter volume in the caudate and lenticular nucleus (Pillay et al. 1998). The third ventricle appears to be enlarged in bipolar (Schlegel and Kretzschmar 1987) but not in unipolar subjects (Coffey et al. 1993).

Most studies of mood disorders have not shown conclusive evidence of generalized brain atrophy (Soares and Innis 2000; Soares and Mann 1997). A meta-analysis of this literature (Elkis et al. 1995), however, found evidence of increased ventricular enlargement in mood disorder subjects, with an effect size that was small in magnitude but statistically significant. This postulated difference in cerebral volume between mood disorder patients and healthy individuals has not been confirmed in most controlled studies conducted to date (Aylward et al. 1994; Coffey et al. 1993; Harvey et al. 1994; Krishnan et al. 1992).

Blood Flow and Metabolism Findings

Brain blood flow and glucose metabolism studies in mood disorder patients have reported similar patterns of abnormalities in unipolar and bipolar mood disorders, primarily involving prefrontal cortical, subcortical, and limbic structures (Soares and Innis 2000). Most single photon emission computed tomography (SPECT) (Ito et al. 1996) and PET cerebral blood flow and glucose metabolism studies (Buchsbaum et al. 1986) in bipolar individuals have shown evidence of hypofrontality. This is similar to what has been reported in unipolar patients (Mayberg et al. 1994). Most studies of temporal lobe blood flow in bipolar patients have suggested abnormalities in this area (Rubin et al. 1995). Some (Mayberg et al. 1994) studies in unipolar patients have reported similar findings. A recent report on bipolar and unipolar depressed subjects (Drevets 1999) found a positive correlation between blood flow in the amygdala and severity of depressive symptoms, with a subsequent decrease in blood flow after treatment with antidepressants. Decreases in blood flow and glucose utilization have been observed in the basal ganglia, primarily in the caudate, in unipolar depression (Baxter et al. 1985; Buchsbaum et al. 1986; Mayberg et al. 1994).

Receptor Imaging Studies

Few neuroimaging studies have investigated the dopaminergic system in bipolar disorder patients. There are suggestions of abnormalities, with a report of increased concentrations of striatal D_2 dopamine receptors (Pearlson et al. 1995) in psychotic compared with nonpsychotic bipolar patients. In euthymic bipolar subjects, there is evidence of increased behavioral response to amphetamine but not of increased amphetamine-stimulated dopamine release or of abnormalities in baseline D_2 striatal binding (Anand et al. 2000), suggesting the presence of enhanced postsynaptic dopamine responsivity in bipolar disorder patients. One PET study found reduced D_1 binding potential in the frontal cortex in medication-free bipolar subjects compared with healthy controls (Suhara et al. 1992), but no significant differences in the striatum.

Neuroimaging investigations of the serotonergic system in mood disorders have started to be conducted in the past few years. A recent study in unipolar and bipolar depressed subjects found decreased density of 5-HT_{1A} receptors in several brain regions (Drevets et al. 1999). Furthermore, this abnormal decrease was greatest in the midbrain raphe. These changes were most pronounced in bipolar or unipolar depressed patients who had a family history of bipolar disorder. Other studies report serotonergic abnormalities in unipolar depressed subjects (Biver et al. 1997), a finding that highlights the dysfunction of this neurotransmitter system in affective disorders.

Magnetic Resonance Spectroscopy Studies

Proton magnetic resonance spectroscopy (MRS) permits in vivo measurement of some molecules and metabolites that can play a role in the pathophysiology of neuropsychiatric disorders. Proton MRS can quantitate brain levels of molecules such as N-acetyl-aspartate (NAA), choline, myoinositol, creatine, and GABA. Decreased levels of NAA have been found in the dorsolateral prefrontal cortex of bipolar disorder subjects (Winsberg et al. 2000), suggesting abnormal neural processes in this brain region. A trend toward increased myoinositol levels was reported in the right dorsolateral prefrontal cortex of lithium-free euthymic bipolar patients (Winsberg et al. 2000). Phosphorus 31 (^{31}P) MRS findings in bipolar subjects are consistent with increased membrane anabolism in the depressed and manic phases of the illness, as measured by the levels of phosphomonoesters and phosphodiesters (Kato et al. 1994). In euthymic bipolar patients, there is evidence of decreased membrane anabolism, at least in the frontal and temporal lobes (Deicken et al. 1995).

Signaling Pathways

The observation that some drugs that act primarily on monoaminergic systems can produce changes in emotional states has led to studies examining the role of these neurotransmitters in mood disorders. Findings that substances such as reserpine, physostigmine, and antidepressants can modulate affect have contributed to hypotheses specifying how neurotransmitter and receptor signaling disturbances produce depressive or manic symptoms. The neurotransmitter and receptor abnormalities that have been identified over the years still do not fully explain the complex clinical presentations of mood disorders. Recently, the focus of this research has shifted to the potential role of second, third, and fourth messengers and transcription factors in the pathophysiology of bipolar disorder as well as to the mechanisms of action of antimanic treatments. We attempt here to briefly review the findings in cell signaling in bipolar disorder with a more detailed approach concerning intracellular abnormalities.

Neurotransmitters

Findings from studies that examined the levels of norepinephrine and its major metabolite, 3-methoxy-4-hydroxyphenylglycol (MHPG), in cerebrospinal fluid (CSF), plasma, and urine in bipolar patients (Manji and Potter 1997) indicate greater excretion and turnover of norepinephrine during depressed states and increased norepinephrine activity during mania. A possible mechanism explaining the increased noradrenergic activity in affective disorders could be a subsensitivity of inhibitory α_2-adrenoreceptors (Manji and Potter 1997). α_2-Adrenoreceptor subsensitivity in depression could account for the blunted growth hormone (GH) response to clonidine (Ansseau et al. 1988) and the results of studies of α_2-adrenoreceptor inhibition of platelet adenylyl cyclase (Kafka and Paul 1986) in this population. It is possible that a subsensitivity of α_2-adrenoreceptors could increase the amount of norepinephrine released at the synaptic terminal—or, alternatively, that greater amounts of norepinephrine at the synaptic cleft might depress α_2-adrenoreceptor activation in affective disorders.

　　The activity of dopamine originating from mesocorticolimbic neurons has been linked to reward and motivational behavior. Deficiencies in dopamine reward circuits appear to be related to anhedonia in animal models of depression (Wilner 1995). CSF levels of the dopamine metabolite homovanillic acid (HVA) are reduced in depression (Manji and Potter 1997) and appear to be elevated in mania (Anand and Charney 2000). Peripheral HVA secretion is also reduced in depression, although it has been found to be increased in psychotic depression (Lykouras et al. 1995). The fact that no abnormalities in dopamine-mediated GH release have been found suggests that D_2 function is preserved in bipolar disorder (Hirschowitz et al. 1986).

There is considerable evidence linking serotonin and mood abnormalities (Oquendo and Mann 2000). However, most available studies have been performed in patients with unipolar major depression. A decrease in serotonin uptake sites in platelets has been reported in bipolar disorder, particularly in bipolar depression (Meltzer et al. 1981). CSF levels of 5-hydroxyindoleacetic acid (5-HIAA), the major metabolite of 5-HT, appear to correlate more closely with suicidal and/or aggressive behavior than with major depression (Goodwin 1986). Moreover, some authors have not found evidence of lower CSF 5-HIAA levels in bipolar patients, even in suicide attempters (Asberg et al. 1987). Genetic studies attempting to link dysfunction of 5-HT receptors or transporter genes with vulnerability for bipolar disorder have found only weak associations thus far (Oquendo and Mann 2000).

GABA is used by at least one-third of all synapses in the human brain; it mediates neurotransmission in key areas involved in mood regulation, such as the striatum, globus pallidus, and cerebral cortex, through interneuronal synapses (Massat et al. 2000). Some animal models of depression show reductions in $GABA_B$ receptors in the frontal cortex (Martin et al. 1989). Postmortem studies have demonstrated decreased activity of glutamic acid decarboxylase, the GABA-synthesizing enzyme, in the frontal and occipital cortices, caudate nucleus, and substantia nigra of depressed subjects (Shiah and Yatham 1998). This might produce reduced GABA activity in this brain region during depressive episodes (Shiah and Yatham 1998). This reduction in GABAergic activity is supported by findings of decreased $GABA_A$ receptor density in the frontal cortex of depressed suicide victims (Cheetham et al. 1988). The action of anticonvulsants as mood stabilizers provides further evidence for GABA's involvement in mood regulation. Chronic administration of valproate, carbamazepine, and lithium decreases GABA turnover and enhances GABAergic neurotransmission (Post et al. 1992). Furthermore, upregulation of $GABA_B$ receptors in the frontal cortex and hippocampus, and downregulation in the hypothalamus, has been shown to be a common feature of chronic use of all mood stabilizers (Motohashi 1992). Lower GABA plasma levels are also present in depressed patients (Prosser et al. 1997), whereas higher plasma GABA levels have a positive correlation with better valproate response in mania (Petty et al. 1996).

G Proteins and Intracellular Messengers

The phospholipid membrane bilayer that defines the limits of all cells plays a crucial role in neurotransmission. Receptors, G proteins, ion channels, and transporters are anchored within this membrane. Cell membrane components have mostly been studied in vivo in red blood cells and platelets (Mallinger 2000), which are thought to approximate brain cell membranes. A membrane's function and permeability are strongly connected with the concentration and distribution of different phospholipids in its bilayer. Briefly, inositol- and amino-phospholipids (e.g., phosphatidylserine, phosphatidylethanolamine, and phosphatidylinositol) are more abundant on the internal surface and are involved in the production of second-messenger components of the phosphatidylinositol intracellular signaling pathway. Choline-phospholipids (e.g., phosphatidylcholine and sphyngomyelin) are more common outside the cell and are associated with membrane fluidity (Mallinger 2000).

In addition to the MRS studies reporting abnormalities in membrane phospholipid turnover in certain brain regions of bipolar patients (see "Magnetic Resonance Spectroscopy Studies" section earlier in this chapter), there is evidence of membrane dysfunction in peripheral tissues. Alterations in the hydrophobic region of red blood cell and lymphocyte membranes have been found in bipolar patients (Pettegrew et al. 1982). Abnormal levels of phosphatydilcholine have been observed in schizophrenia and in manic patients (Hitzemann et al. 1986). Abnormalities in the levels of phosphatidylcholine can potentially alter membrane fluidity and function, including Na^+-Li^+ countertransport activity (Mallinger 2000). Although their causes are still unknown, phosphatydilcholine anomalies might represent abnormal membrane processes in bipolar subjects. Studies of lithium's effects in cell membranes are discussed below.

The effectiveness of receptor-neurotransmitter coupling in producing a specific cellular response relies on the ability of a transduction system to translate this membrane signal into the intracellular environment. Most neurotransmitters and neuromodulators are coupled to a G protein system to promote intracellular effects. G proteins have multiple subunits (α, β, and γ) that can stimulate (G_s) or inhibit (G_i) different intracellular enzymatic systems, such as adenylyl cyclase, which produces cyclic adenosine 3',5'-monophosphate (cAMP), and phospholipase C, which produces diacylglycerol. These second messengers, cAMP and diacylglycerol, are responsible for activating protein kinases A and C, respectively. When activated, protein kinases phosphorylate various substrate proteins. As a result, these kinases regulate metabolic functions within the cell and, eventually, activate gene transcription factors responsible for long-lasting modifications of cellular status (Soares and Mallinger 2000).

Postmortem studies of G protein levels in brains of bipolar disorder patients have shown abnormalities such as increased levels of the long-spliced variant of $G_s\alpha$ in frontal, temporal, and occipital cortices and higher levels of the short variant in the hippocampus and caudate nucleus (Warsh 2000). Moreover, $G\alpha_{q/11}$ levels were observed to be higher only in the occipital cortex of bipolar disorder patients (Mathews et al. 1997). On the other hand, no abnormalities of other G protein subunits have been detected (Friedman and Wang 1996; Young et al. 1993). In peripheral cells, there have been reports of increased levels of specific $G_s\alpha$ subtypes in unmedicated bipolar patients (Manji et al. 1995). Warsh (2000) postulated that increased levels of certain $G_s\alpha$ subtypes may be explained by alterations of posttranslational processes, because there is no evidence of increased $G_s\alpha$ mRNA in the brain regions where higher $G_s\alpha$ levels have been reported (Young et al. 1996). In depressed bipolar subjects, decreased levels of $G_s\alpha$ and $G_i\alpha$ in leukocytes have been observed (Avissar et al. 1997).

There is compelling evidence suggesting abnormalities in G protein function and G protein concentrations in bipolar patients. Increased G protein function was found in leukocytes of unmedicated manic patients compared with lithium-treated euthymic bipolar patients and healthy controls (Schreiber et al. 1991). In postmortem studies, investigations have provided evidence of increased $G_s\alpha$-coupled adenylyl cyclase activity in the temporal and occipital cortices (Young et al. 1993). $G\alpha_{q/11}$ binding was also significantly higher in the frontal cortex of postmortem brains from bipolar patients (Friedman and Wang 1996). Given that $G_s\alpha$ and $G\alpha_{q/11}$ couple to different second-messenger systems (cAMP and phosphoinositol, respectively), these abnormalities could lead to important downstream effects on intracellular signaling in the brains of bipolar patients.

Initial investigations focused on plasma, CSF, and intracellular levels of cAMP. Early studies showed that the levels of cAMP in these biological systems appear to be normal in mood disorder patients during different mood states (Maj et al. 1984). However, varying results have been obtained, including increases (Kay et al. 1993) and decreases (Ebstein et al. 1988) in stimulated adenylyl cyclase activity in peripheral cells of bipolar patients compared with healthy controls. Reductions in receptor-stimulated cAMP response to β-adrenergic stimulation have been demonstrated in depressed patients (Mann et al. 1985). In postmortem studies, however, forskolin-stimulated cAMP production was significantly increased in the temporal and occipital cortices of bipolar patients (Young et al. 1993). Finally, cAMP-dependent phosphorylation also appears to be increased in bipolar disorder. Incorporation of phosphorus 32 (^{32}P) in platelets and phosphorylation of Rap1, a small protein whose intracellular function is as yet unknown, are increased in medication-free euthymic bipolar patients (Perez et al. 1995).

More recent evidence implicates the phosphatidylinositol (PI) pathway in bipolar disorder. Platelet membranes from manic patients have increased phosphatidylinositol 4,5-bisphosphate (PIP$_2$) levels (Brown et al. 1993). These results suggest a hyperfunctional state in the PI pathway during the manic state, which could be reversed with mood normalization and/or lithium treatment (Soares and Mallinger 2000). The intracellular level of myoinositol, a precursor in the PI pathway, appears to be relevant to the pathophysiology of mood disorders. Postmortem studies have indicated lower levels of myoinositol (Shimon et al. 1997) in the frontal cortex of bipolar patients, although the activity of the enzyme inositol monophosphatase has been reported to be normal (Shimon et al. 1997). The function of phospholipase C (PLC) has also been found to be normal in the frontal, temporal, and occipital cortices in postmortem studies of bipolar patients (Mathews et al. 1997).

Abnormalities reported in the cAMP and PI signaling systems in bipolar disorder may also be present in downstream levels of these pathways (i.e., protein kinases). Alterations in cAMP-dependent protein kinase (PKA) levels and function could provide additional evidence of elevated cAMP activity in bipolar patients. Decreased levels of regulatory subunits of PKA have been observed in postmortem brains of bipolar disorder patients (Rahman et al. 1997). It is postulated that the loss of these inhibitory regulatory units might increase PKA activity (Warsh 2000). Supporting this hypothesis, one postmortem study reported enhanced PKA catalytic activity in the temporal cortex of bipolar patients (Fields et al. 1999). In vivo studies of platelets likewise have provided evidence of abnormal cAMP-stimulated endogenous phosphorylation in euthymic bipolar patients (Perez et al. 1995). PKA plays an important role in intracellular processes; it is responsible for almost all cAMP-mediated phosphorylation reactions. Furthermore, the activity of PKA appears to be influenced by antidepressants, electroconvulsive therapy (ECT), and mood stabilizers (Nestler et al. 1989).

There is also evidence for protein kinase C (PKC) abnormalities in bipolar disorder. Increased membrane-associated PKC activity in platelets was reported in medication-free manic bipolar patients, but not in control subjects or those with schizophrenia (Friedman et al. 1993). In postmortem studies of bipolar subjects compared with healthy control subjects, higher PKC activity; higher levels of α, γ, and ε PKC isozymes; and reduced levels of ε PKC in the frontal cortex were reported (Wang and Friedman 1996). This increased PKC activity is inhibited by the action of mood stabilizers (Hahn and Friedman 1999). In summary, there is compelling evidence of upregulated PKA and PKC signaling pathways in bipolar patients.

Several G protein–coupled receptors can activate the hydrolysis of membrane phospholipids in the PI pathway. In this process, PIP_2 is catalyzed by the action of PLC to generate diacylglycerol (DAG) and inositol trisphosphate (IP_3). Both DAG (which activates the phosphorylating action of PKC) and IP_3 regulate the level of intracellular calcium (Hahn and Friedman 1999). Increased baseline calcium levels were found in peripheral cells of medication-free bipolar patients (Dubovsky et al. 1994). Calcium response to stimulation was also found to be increased in unmedicated bipolar subjects (van Calker et al. 1993) but decreased in lithium-treated euthymic patients (Forstner et al. 1994). Increased intracellular calcium function is consistent with the hypothesis of a hyperactive PI pathway in bipolar disorders.

The long-lasting actions of psychiatric medications involve modifications of the regulation and expression of target genes. Several transcription factors—such as Fos, Jun, and cAMP response element binding protein (CREB)—have been identified thus far, and they play key roles in the long-term effects of antidepressants and mood stabilizers.

Psychopharmacology

Although lithium salt has been used in a variety of psychiatric conditions, its effectiveness and specificity in the treatment of bipolar mood disorder has been extensively established in the literature. Thus, a clearer understanding of the specific actions of this ion in the brain could provide important insights into the pathophysiology of bipolar disorder.

Lithium has important effects on various neurotransmitter systems, as has been extensively reviewed elsewhere (Lenox and Hahn 2000). In brief, it has been found to increase dopamine turnover and decrease its formation (Engel and Berggren 1980), and to enhance serotonergic transmission by acutely increasing the amount of 5-HT release (Hotta and Yamawaki 1988). Lithium may have bimodal effects on norepinephrine, initially lowering norepinephrine-stimulated β-adrenergic receptor function and later increasing norepinephrine release through α_2 autoreceptor effects (Lenox and Hahn 2000). Lithium and valproate also appear to enhance GABA function (Motohashi 1992). Glutamate function increases in response to acute treatment (Hokin et al. 1996) but decreases with chronic lithium use (Dixon and Hokin 1998).

Lithium appears to decrease receptor-coupled activation of the cAMP pathway through inhibition of β-adrenergic-stimulated adenylyl cyclase activity (Newman et al. 1983). Although lithium reduces receptor-coupled cAMP accumulation, there is evidence that basal cAMP levels increase with lithium treatment. It has been postulated that lithium can uncouple $G\alpha_i$ inhibition of adenylyl cyclase, leading to enhanced cAMP production (Lenox and Hahn 2000). This bimodal model of lithium's action has been proposed to partially explain its efficacy in manic and depressive phases. Consistent with higher levels of cAMP after lithium use, postmortem studies have also shown increased PKA activity in the temporal lobe (Fields et al. 1999).

Lithium is a potent and noncompetitive inhibitor of two important enzymes of the PI cycle: inositol-1-phosphatase and polyphosphatase-1-phosphatase (Nahorski et al. 1991). Inhibition of these enzymes causes a depletion of free inositol and consequent reduction of the resynthesis of PI cycle components, possibly leading to reductions in specific intracellular messengers (Ikonomov and Manji 1999). On the basis of lithium's noncompetitive profile, it has been postulated that lithium's effects are most dramatic in neurons with the highest rates of enzymatic activity (i.e., overactive neural circuits with higher firing rates). Lithium-induced alterations in PI signaling could trigger more longlasting events through PKC-mediated pathways and modulation of gene expression.

Indeed, lithium has complex actions on PKC function. A considerable amount of evidence suggests that chronic lithium administration decreases specific PKC isozymes in the frontal cortex and hippocampus (Manji et al. 1999). In a recent study, lithium was found to decrease levels of cytosolic PKC-α and membrane PIP_2 in platelets of bipolar patients (Soares et al. 2000). One of the most prominent PKC substrates in the brain is the myristolated alanine-rich C kinase substrate (MARCKS). This protein is involved in several intracellular processes, including modulation of synaptic neuroplasticity (Ikonomov and Manji 1999). After 4 weeks of lithium treatment, MARCKS expression was found to be significantly decreased in the hippocampus (Watson and Lenox 1996). Moreover, a recent report highlights the importance of PKC activation in lithium's effects on specific transcription factors (G. Chen et al. 2000).

Lithium regulates gene expression through diverse nuclear transcriptional factors (Lenox and Hahn 2000). Changes in the expression of the immediate-early gene products Fos and Jun have been found after lithium use (Yuan et al. 1999), with differential effects present in specific brain regions and cell types (Lenox and Hahn 2000). These two transcription factors form a heterodimer that binds to an activator protein-1

(AP-1) complex of target genes. Several genes are regulated by AP-1 binding, including genes that encode specific neurotransmitters and neuropeptides, certain membrane receptors, and cytoskeletal restructuring elements (G. Chen et al. 1999). It is postulated that lithium can increase (Manji et al. 1999) or attenuate (Jope and Song 1997) AP-1 DNA binding activity, depending on the level of activation of the genes involved (Lenox and Hahn 2000). Lithium appears to reduce the expression of transcription factor CREB in certain brain areas (B. Chen et al. 1999) and to increase it in others (Ozaki and Chuang 1997), but the relevance of these findings remains unclear.

It was recently demonstrated that lithium can protect neurons from apoptosis induced by N-methyl-D-aspartate (NMDA)–mediated excitotoxicity (Nonaka et al. 1998), among other insults. This neuroprotective effect became apparent only after chronic treatment. It is known that certain neurotrophic factors can inhibit apoptosis and cell injury in response to various insults. The expression of one of these neurotrophic factors (Bcl-2) increases in certain brain regions after chronic lithium treatment (Manji et al. 1999). MRS findings have provided in vivo evidence of lithium's protective action in human subjects (Moore et al. 2000). Lithium treatment increased N-acetylaspartate, a putative marker of neuronal viability, in several brain regions of bipolar patients. Long-term modulation of gene expression by lithium may be related to lithium's neuroprotective effects, although it is not yet clear what role neuroprotection might play in mood stabilization.

The long-lasting mood-stabilizing effects of valproate also involve activation of several transcription factors. An increase of AP-1 DNA binding activity was demonstrated in response to valproate administration (G. Chen et al. 1999). Like lithium, valproate increases the regional expression of CREB and Fos, although the regions at which these increases occur differ for lithium and valproate in rat brain (B. Chen et al. 1999). On the other hand, valproate appears to inhibit PKC signaling (Manji et al. 1996) in a manner similar to lithium, whereas carbamazepine appears to inhibit cAMP pathways (Manji et al. 1996). These differences in the intracellular effects of mood stabilizers could explain the diverse profiles and therapeutic actions of lithium, carbamazepine, and valproate.

Conclusions

Evidence supports the involvement of discrete brain regions and circuits in mood regulation—in particular, the brain pathways that interconnect prefrontal cortex, striatum, pallidum, thalamus, and limbic structures. Although bipolar and unipolar mood disorders apparently share some biological characteristics, there are specific findings of abnormalities in signal transduction pathways, including intracellular messengers, protein kinase activity, G protein levels, and gene expression, that are unique to bipolar disorders. The actions of lithium and anticonvulsants on intracellular signaling pathways provide a new paradigm for novel pharmacological interventions. On the basis of these findings, new approaches are being undertaken that attempt to modulate specific steps in these pathways (e.g., the use of PKC or inositol-uptake inhibitors [Belmaker and Yaroslavsky 2000]). These developments could ultimately produce substantial advances in the pharmacological treatment of bipolar patients.

References

Altshuler LL, Conrad A, Hauser P, et al: Reduction of temporal lobe volume in bipolar disorder: a preliminary report of magnetic resonance imaging. Arch Gen Psychiatry 48:482–483, 1991

Anand A, Charney DS: Abnormalities in catecholamines and pathophysiology of bipolar disorder, in Bipolar Disorders: Basic Mechanisms and Therapeutic Implications. Edited by Soares JC, Gershon S. New York, Marcel Dekker, 2000, pp 59–94

Anand A, Verhoeff P, Seneca N, et al: Brain SPECT imaging of amphetamine-induced dopamine release in euthymic bipolar disorder patients. Am J Psychiatry 157:1108–1114, 2000

Ansseau M, Von Frenckell R, Cerfontaine JL, et al: Blunted response of growth hormone to clonidine and apomorphine in endogenous depression. Br J Psychiatry 153:65–71, 1988

Asberg M, Schalling D, Traskman-Bendz L, et al: Psychobiology of suicide, impulsivity, and related phenomena, in Psychopharmacology: The Third Generation of Progress. Edited by Meltzer HY. New York, Raven, 1987, pp 655–668

Avissar S, Nechamkin Y, Barki-Harrington L, et al: Differential G protein measures in mononuclear leukocytes of patients with bipolar mood disorder are state dependent. J Affect Disord 43:85–93, 1997

Aylward EH, Roberts-Twillie JV, Barta PE, et al: Basal ganglia volumes and white matter hyperintensities in patients with bipolar disorder. Am J Psychiatry 151:687–693, 1994

Baxter LR Jr, Phelps ME, Mazziotta JC, et al: Cerebral metabolic rates for glucose in mood disorders: studies with positron emission tomography and fluorodeoxyglucose F 18. Arch Gen Psychiatry 42:441–447, 1985

Belmaker RH, Yaroslavsky Y: Perspectives for new pharmacological interventions, in Bipolar Disorders: Basic Mechanisms and Therapeutic Implications. Edited by Soares JC, Gershon S. New York, Marcel Dekker, 2000, pp 507–528

Benes FM, Kwok EW, Vincent SL, et al: A reduction of nonpyramidal cells in sector CA2 of schizophrenics and manic depressives. Biol Psychiatry 44:88–97, 1998

Biver F, Wikler D, Lotstra F, et al: Serotonin 5-HT2 receptor imaging in major depression: focal changes in orbito-insular cortex. Br J Psychiatry 171:444–448, 1997

Brown AS, Mallinger AG, Renbaum LC: Elevated platelet membrane phosphatidylinositol-4,5-bisphosphate in bipolar mania. Am J Psychiatry 150:1252–1254, 1993

Buchsbaum MS, Wu J, DeLisi LE, et al: Frontal cortex and basal ganglia metabolic rates assessed by positron emission tomography with [18F]2-deoxyglucose in affective illness. J Affect Disord 10:137–152, 1986

Cheetham SC, Crompton MR, Katona CL, et al: Brain GABAA/benzodiazepine binding sites and glutamic acid decarboxylase activity in depressed suicide victims. Brain Res 460:114–123, 1988

Chen B, Wang JF, Hill BC, et al: Lithium and valproate differentially regulate brain regional expression of phosphorylated CREB and c-fos. Brain Res Mol Brain Res 70:45–53, 1999

Chen G, Yuan PX, Jiang YM, et al: Valproate robustly enhances AP-1 mediated gene expression. Brain Res Mol Brain Res 64:52–58, 1999

Chen G, Masana MI, Manji HK: Lithium regulates PKC-mediated intracellular cross-talk and gene expression in the CNS in vivo. Bipolar Disord 2 (3 pt 2):217–236, 2000

Coffey CE, Wilkinson WE, Weiner RD, et al: Quantitative cerebral anatomy in depression: a controlled magnetic resonance imaging study. Arch Gen Psychiatry 50:7–16, 1993

Coryell W, Endicott J, Maser JD, et al: Long-term stability of polarity distinctions in the affective disorders. Am J Psychiatry 152:385–390, 1995

Deicken RF, Fein G, Weiner MW: Abnormal frontal lobe phosphorous metabolism in bipolar disorder. Am J Psychiatry 152:915–918, 1995

Dewan MJ, Haldipur CV, Lane EE, et al: Bipolar affective disorder, I: comprehensive quantitative computed tomography. Acta Psychiatr Scand 77:670–676, 1988

Dixon JF, Hokin LE: Lithium acutely inhibits and chronically up-regulates and stabilizes glutamate uptake by presynaptic nerve endings in mouse cerebral cortex. Proc Natl Acad Sci U S A 95:8363–8368, 1998

Drevets WC: Prefrontal cortical-amygdalar metabolism in major depression. Ann N Y Acad Sci 877:614–637, 1999

Drevets WC, Price JL, Simpson JR Jr, et al: Subgenual prefrontal cortex abnormalities in mood disorders. Nature 386:824–827, 1997

Drevets WC, Ongur D, Price JL: Neuroimaging abnormalities in the sub-genual prefrontal cortex—implications for the pathophysiology of familial mood disorders. Mol Psychiatry 3:220–226, 1998

Drevets WC, Frank E, Price JC, et al: PET imaging of serotonin 1A receptor binding in depression. Biol Psychiatry 46:1375–1387, 1999

Dubovsky SL, Thomas M, Hijazi A, et al: Intracellular calcium signalling in peripheral cells of patients with bipolar affective disorder. Eur Arch Psychiatry Clin Neurosci 243:229–234, 1994

Ebstein RP, Lerer B, Shapira B, et al: Cyclic AMP second messenger amplification in depression. Br J Psychiatry 152:665–669, 1988

Elkis H, Friedman L, Wise A, et al: Meta-analyses of studies of ventricular enlargement and cortical sulcal prominence in mood disorders. Comparisons with controls or patients with schizophrenia. Arch Gen Psychiatry 52:735–746, 1995

Engel J, Berggren U: Effects of lithium on behaviour and central monoamines. Acta Psychiatr Scand Suppl 280:133–143, 1980

Fields A, Li PP, Kish SJ, et al: Increased cyclic AMP-dependent protein kinase activity in postmortem brain from patients with bipolar affective disorder. J Neurochem 73:1704–1710, 1999

Forstner U, Bohus M, Gebicke-Harter PJ, et al: Decreased agonist-stimulated Ca2+ response in neutrophils from patients under chronic lithium therapy. Eur Arch Psychiatry Clin Neurosci 243:240–243, 1994

Friedman E, Wang HY: Receptor-mediated activation of G proteins is increased in postmortem brains of bipolar affective disorder subjects. J Neurochem 67:1145–1152, 1996

Friedman E, Hoau-Yan-Wang, Levinson D, et al: Altered platelet protein kinase C activity in bipolar affective disorder, manic episode. Biol Psychiatry 33:520–525, 1993

Goodwin FK: Suicide, aggression, and depression. A theoretical framework for future research. Ann N Y Acad Sci 487:351–355, 1986

Hahn CG, Friedman E: Abnormalities in protein kinase C signaling and the pathophysiology of bipolar disorder. Bipolar Disord 1:81–86, 1999

Harvey I, Persaud R, Ron MA, et al: Volumetric MRI measurements in bipolars compared with schizophrenics and healthy controls. Psychol Med 24:689–699, 1994

Hirschowitz J, Zemlan FP, Hitzemann RJ, et al: Growth hormone response to apomorphine and diagnosis: a comparison of three diagnostic systems. Biol Psychiatry 21:445–454, 1986

Hitzemann RJ, Hirschowitz J, Garver DL: On the physical properties of red cell ghost membranes in the affective disorders and psychoses: a fluorescence polarization study. J Affect Disord 10:227–232, 1986

Hokin LE, Dixon JF, Los GV: A novel action of lithium: stimulation of glutamate release and inositol 1,4,5 trisphosphate accumulation via activation of the N-methyl D-aspartate receptor in monkey and mouse cerebral cortex slices. Adv Enzyme Regul 36:229–244, 1996

Hotta I, Yamawaki S: Possible involvement of presynaptic 5-HT autoreceptors in effect of lithium on 5-HT release in hippocampus of rat. Neuropharmacology 27:987–992, 1988

Husain MM, McDonald WM, Doraiswamy PM, et al: A magnetic resonance imaging study of putamen nuclei in major depression. Psychiatry Res 40:95–99, 1991

Ikonomov OC, Manji HK: Molecular mechanisms underlying mood stabilization in manic-depressive illness: the phenotype challenge. Am J Psychiatry 156:1506–1514, 1999

Ito H, Kawashima R, Awata S, et al: Hypoperfusion in the limbic system and prefrontal cortex in depression: SPECT with anatomic standardization technique. J Nucl Med 37:410–414, 1996

Jope RS, Song L: AP-1 and NF-kappaB stimulated by carbachol in human neuroblastoma SH-SY5Y cells are differentially sensitive to inhibition by lithium. Brain Res Mol Brain Res 50:171–180, 1997

Kafka MS, Paul SM: Platelet alpha 2-adrenergic receptors in depression. Arch Gen Psychiatry 43:91–95, 1986

Kato T, Shioiri T, Murashita J, et al: Phosphorus-31 magnetic resonance spectroscopy and ventricular enlargement in bipolar disorder. Psychiatry Res 55:41–50, 1994

Kay G, Sargeant M, McGuffin P: The lymphoblast beta-adrenergic receptor in bipolar depressed patients: characterization and down-regulation. J Affect Disord 27:163–172, 1993

Krishnan KR, McDonald WM, Escalona PR, et al: Magnetic resonance imaging of the caudate nuclei in depression. Preliminary observations. Arch Gen Psychiatry 49:553–557, 1992

Lenox RH, Hahn CG: Overview of the mechanism of action of lithium in the brain: fifty-year update. J Clin Psychiatry 61 (suppl 9):5–15, 2000

Lykouras L, Markianos M, Hatzimanolis J, et al: Association of biogenic amine metabolites with symptomatology in delusional (psychotic) and nondelusional depressed patients. Prog Neuropsychopharmacol Biol Psychiatry 19:877–887, 1995

Maj M, Ariano MG, Arena F, et al: Plasma cortisol, catecholamine and cyclic AMP levels, response to dexamethasone suppression test and platelet MAO activity in manic-depressive patients: a longitudinal study. Neuropsychobiology 11:168–173, 1984

Mallinger AG: Cell membrane abnormalities in bipolar disorder, in Bipolar Disorders: Basic Mechanisms and Therapeutic Implications. Edited by Soares JC, Gershon S. New York, Marcel Dekker, 2000, pp 167–177

Manji HK, Potter WZ: Monoaminergic systems, in Bipolar Disorder: Biological Models and Their Clinical Application. Edited by Young LT, Joffe RT. New York, Marcel Dekker, 1997, pp 1–40

Manji HK, Chen G, Shimon H, et al: Guanine nucleotide-binding proteins in bipolar affective disorder. Effects of long-term lithium treatment. Arch Gen Psychiatry 52:135–144, 1995

Manji HK, Chen G, Hsiao JK, et al: Regulation of signal transduction pathways by mood-stabilizing agents: implications for the delayed onset of therapeutic efficacy. J Clin Psychiatry 57 (suppl 13):34–46, 1996

Manji HK, Bebchuk JM, Moore GJ, et al: Modulation of CNS signal transduction pathways and gene expression by mood-stabilizing agents: therapeutic implications. J Clin Psychiatry 60 (suppl 2):27–39, 1999

Mann JJ, Brown RP, Halper JP, et al: Reduced sensitivity of lymphocyte beta-adrenergic receptors in patients with endogenous depression and psychomotor agitation. N Engl J Med 313:715–720, 1985

Martin P, Pichat P, Massol J, et al: Decreased GABA B receptors in helpless rats: reversal by tricyclic antidepressants. Neuropsychobiology 22:220–224, 1989

Massat I, Souery D, Mendlewicz J, et al: The GABAergic hypothesis of mood disorder, in Bipolar Disorders: Basic Mechanisms and Therapeutic Implications. Edited by Soares JC, Gershon S. New York, Marcel Dekker, 2000, pp 143–165

Mathews R, Li PP, Young LT, et al: Increased G alpha q/11 immunoreactivity in postmortem occipital cortex from patients with bipolar affective disorder. Biol Psychiatry 41:649–656, 1997

Mayberg HS, Starkstein SE, Peyser CE, et al: Paralimbic frontal lobe hypometabolism in depression associated with Huntington's disease. Neurology 42: 1791–1797, 1992

Mayberg HS, Lewis PJ, Regenold W, et al: Paralimbic hypoperfusion in unipolar depression. J Nucl Med 35:929–934, 1994

Meltzer HY, Ramesh CA, Arora RC, et al: Serotonin uptake in blood platelets of psychiatric patients. Arch Gen Psychiatry 38:1322–1326, 1981

Moore GJ, Bebchuk JM, Hasanat K, et al: Lithium increases N-acetyl-aspartate in the human brain: in vivo evidence in support of bcl-2's neurotrophic effects? Biol Psychiatry 48:1–8, 2000

Motohashi N: GABA receptor alterations after chronic lithium administration. Comparison with carbamazepine and sodium valproate. Prog Neuropsychopharmacol Biol Psychiatry 16:571–579, 1992

Nahorski SR, Ragan CI, Challiss RA: Lithium and the phosphoinositide cycle: an example of uncompetitive inhibition and its pharmacological consequences. Trends Pharmacol Sci 12:297–303, 1991

Nestler EJ, Terwilliger RZ, Duman RS: Chronic antidepressant administration alters the subcellular distribution of cyclic AMP-dependent protein kinase in rat frontal cortex. J Neurochem 53:1644–1647, 1989

Newman M, Klein E, Birmaher B, et al: Lithium at therapeutic concentrations inhibits human brain noradrenaline-sensitive cyclic AMP accumulation. Brain Res 278:380–381, 1983

Nonaka S, Hough CJ, Chuang DM: Chronic lithium treatment robustly protects neurons in the central nervous system against excitotoxicity by inhibiting N-methyl-D-aspartate receptor-mediated calcium influx. Proc Natl Acad Sci U S A 95:2642–2647, 1998

Ongur D, Drevets WC, Price JL: Glial reduction in the subgenual prefrontal cortex in mood disorders. Proc Natl Acad Sci U S A 95:13290–13295, 1998

Oquendo MA, Mann JJ: Serotonergic dysfunction in mood disorder, in Bipolar Disorders: Basic Mechanisms and Therapeutic Implications. Edited by Soares JC, Gershon S. New York, Marcel Dekker, 2000, pp 121–142

Ozaki N, Chuang DM: Lithium increases transcription factor binding to AP-1 and cyclic AMP-responsive element in cultured neurons and rat brain. J Neurochem 69:2336–2344, 1997

Paykel ES: Handbook of Affective Disorders, 2nd Edition. New York, Guilford, 1992

Pearlson GD, Wong DF, Tune LE, et al: In vivo D_2 dopamine receptor density in psychotic and nonpsychotic patients with bipolar disorder. Arch Gen Psychiatry 52:471–477, 1995

Pearlson GD, Barta PE, Powers RE, et al: Ziskind-Somerfeld Research Award 1996. Medial and superior temporal gyral volumes and cerebral asymmetry in schizophrenia versus bipolar disorder. Biol Psychiatry 41:1–14, 1997

Perez J, Zanardi R, Mori S, et al: Abnormalities of cAMP-dependent endogenous phosphorylation in platelets from patients with bipolar disorder. Am J Psychiatry 152:1204–1206, 1995

Pettegrew JW, Nichols JS, Minshew NJ, et al: Membrane biophysical studies of lymphocytes and erythrocytes in manic-depressive illness. J Affect Disord 4:237–247, 1982

Petty F, Rush AJ, Davis JM, et al: Plasma GABA predicts acute response to divalproex in mania. Biol Psychiatry 39:278–284, 1996

Pillay SS, Renshaw PF, Bonello CM, et al: A quantitative magnetic resonance imaging study of caudate and lenticular nucleus gray matter volume in primary unipolar major depression: relationship to treatment response and clinical severity. Psychiatry Res 84:61–74, 1998

Post RM, Weiss SR, Chuang DM: Mechanisms of action of anticonvulsants in affective disorders: comparisons with lithium. J Clin Psychopharmacol 12 (1 suppl):23S–35S, 1992

Prosser J, Hughes CW, Sheikha S, et al: Plasma GABA in children and adolescents with mood, behavior, and comorbid mood and behavior disorders: a preliminary study. J Child Adolesc Psychopharmacol 7:181–199, 1997

Rahman S, Li PP, Young LT, et al: Reduced [3H]cyclic AMP binding in postmortem brain from subjects with bipolar affective disorder. J Neurochem 68: 297–304, 1997

Rajkowska G, Selemon LD, Goldman-Rakic PS: Marked glial neuropathology in prefrontal cortex distinguishes bipolar disorder from schizophrenia (abstract). Schizophr Res 24:41, 1997

Rajkowska G, Miguel-Hidalgo JJ, Wei J, et al: Morphometric evidence for neuronal and glial prefrontal cell pathology in major depression. Biol Psychiatry 45:1085–1098, 1999

Rubin E, Sackeim HA, Prohovnik I, et al: Regional cerebral blood flow in mood disorders, IV: comparison of mania and depression. Psychiatry Res 61:1–10, 1995

Sax KW, Strakowski SM, Zimmerman ME, et al: Frontosubcortical neuroanatomy and the continuous performance test in mania. Am J Psychiatry 156: 139–141, 1999

Schlegel S, Kretzschmar K: Computed tomography in affective disorders, part I: ventricular and sulcal measurements. Biol Psychiatry 22:4–14, 1987

Schreiber G, Avissar S, Danon A, et al: Hyperfunctional G proteins in mononuclear leukocytes of patients with mania. Biol Psychiatry 29:273–280, 1991

Shiah IS, Yatham LN: GABA function in mood disorders: an update and critical review. Life Sci 63:1289–1303, 1998

Shimon H, Agam G, Belmaker RH, et al: Reduced frontal cortex inositol levels in postmortem brain of suicide victims and patients with bipolar disorder. Am J Psychiatry 154:1148–1150, 1997

Soares JC, Innis RB: Brain imaging findings in bipolar disorder, in Bipolar Disorders: Basic Mechanisms and Therapeutic Implications. Edited by Soares JC, Gershon S. New York, Marcel Dekker, 2000, pp 227–252

Soares JC, Mallinger AG: Intracellular signal transduction dysfunction in bipolar disorder, in Bipolar Disorders: Basic Mechanisms and Therapeutic Implications. Edited by Soares JC, Gershon S. New York, Marcel Dekker, 2000, pp 179–200

Soares JC, Mann JJ: The anatomy of mood disorders—review of structural neuroimaging studies. Biol Psychiatry 41:86–106, 1997

Soares JC, Chen G, Dippold CS, et al: Concurrent measures of protein kinase C and phosphoinositides in lithium-treated bipolar patients and healthy individuals: a preliminary study. Psychiatry Res 95:109–118, 2000

Strakowski SM, DelBello MP, Sax KW, et al: Brain magnetic resonance imaging of structural abnormalities in bipolar disorder. Arch Gen Psychiatry 56: 254–260, 1999

Suhara T, Nakayama K, Inoue O, et al: D1 dopamine receptor binding in mood disorders measured by positron emission tomography. Psychopharmacology (Berl) 106:14–18, 1992

Swayze VW 2nd, Andreasen NC, Alliger RJ, et al: Subcortical and temporal structures in affective disorder and schizophrenia: a magnetic resonance imaging study. Biol Psychiatry 31:221–240, 1992

van Calker D, Forstner U, Bohus M, et al: Increased sensitivity to agonist stimulation of the Ca2+ response in neutrophils of manic-depressive patients: effect of lithium therapy. Neuropsychobiology 27:180–183, 1993

Wang HY, Friedman E: Enhanced protein kinase C activity and translocation in bipolar affective disorder brains. Biol Psychiatry 40:568–575, 1996

Warsh JJ: Postmortem brain studies in bipolar disorder, in Bipolar Disorders: Basic Mechanisms and Therapeutic Implications. Edited by Soares JC, Gershon S. New York, Marcel Dekker, 2000, pp 201–226

Watson DG, Lenox RH: Chronic lithium-induced down-regulation of MARCKS in immortalized hippocampal cells: potentiation by muscarinic receptor activation. J Neurochem 67:767–777, 1996

Weissman MM, Leaf PJ, Tischler GL, et al: Affective disorders in five United States communities. Psychol Med 18:141–153, 1988

Wilner P: Dopaminergic mechanisms in depression and mania, in Psychopharmacology: The Fourth Generation of Progress. Edited by Kupfer DJ. New York, Raven, 1995, pp 921–931

Winsberg ME, Sachs N, Tate DL, et al: Decreased dorsolateral prefrontal N-acetyl aspartate in bipolar disorder. Biol Psychiatry 47:475–481, 2000

Young LT, Li PP, Kish SJ, et al: Cerebral cortex Gs alpha protein levels and forskolin-stimulated cyclic AMP formation are increased in bipolar affective disorder. J Neurochem 61:890–898, 1993

Young LT, Asghari V, Li PP, et al: Stimulatory G-protein alpha-subunit mRNA levels are not increased in autopsied cerebral cortex from patients with bipolar disorder. Brain Res Mol Brain Res 42:45–50, 1996

Yuan P, Chen G, Manji HK: Lithium activates the c-Jun NH2-terminal kinases in vitro and in the CNS in vivo. J Neurochem 73:2299–2309, 1999

CHAPTER 8

Neural Circuitry and Signaling in Dementia and Alzheimer's Disease

Ralph A. Nixon, M.D., Ph.D.

Clinical Presentation

Dementia, as defined in DSM-IV-TR (American Psychiatric Association 2000), is an impairment of memory accompanied by aphasia, apraxia, agnosia, or disturbed executive functioning. These cognitive deficits develop gradually, progress over time, and represent a decline in level of functioning sufficient to impair social or occupational performance significantly. The deficits cannot be explained by other Axis I disorders or delirium.

Although dozens of disorders lead to dementia, the majority of cases of dementia (>90%) are accounted for by only a handful of conditions. Alzheimer's disease (AD) and related disorders account for more than 50% of all cases of dementia, vascular dementia and stroke account for 15%–20% of cases, and Parkinson's disease and brain injury account for about 8% and 5%, respectively. The cognitive symptoms observed in these degenerative states have distinctive features, reflecting both the different sites involved and the differing severities of neuropathology, although the patterns of cognitive impairment often significantly overlap (Benson 1993; Cummings 1990).

One useful framework for distinguishing behavioral and cognitive features of various dementia syndromes is based on whether neurodegeneration is predominantly in the cortex, as in dementia of the Alzheimer's type (DAT), or in the subcortical nuclei, as in Huntington's disease. Because both cortical and subcortical structures usually

I thank Lucy Morales for assistance in preparing this manuscript. Space limitations precluded citation of primary references for many findings discussed here. Reviews have been cited that contain these original references.

become involved, it should be emphasized that this cortical-subcortical distinction is rarely absolute. In cortical dementia, memory impairment is severe and appears to result from ineffective *consolidation* or *storage* of new information. Individuals with cortical dementia exhibit only modest improvement in the acquisition of information over repeated learning trials, tend to recall only the most frequently presented information, and forget this information over time. By contrast, in Huntington's disease, memory disturbance is more moderate and reflects greater deficits in information *retrieval*. Noncognitive signs and symptoms are also helpful in distinguishing between these two general patterns of dementing disorders. Cortical dementia may include deficits in language, semantic knowledge (i.e., aphasia), abstract reasoning, and other executive functions. In subcortical dementias, aphasias are uncommon but attentional dysfunction, problem-solving deficits, and psychomotor slowing are prominent. Motor abnormalities, related to the degeneration of specific subcortical structures, are often diagnostic. Depression, accompanied by psychomotor retardation, is usually prominent. Because of strong subcortical projections to the frontal cortex, frontal lobe symptoms are a characteristic feature of subcortical dementia but are also a prominent feature of primary frontal dementias and may develop in frontotemporal dementias, including AD.

As the most common of the dementias, AD has been intensively investigated over the past two decades. In this chapter I focus on advances in understanding the clinical symptoms, neuropathology, genetics, and pathophysiology of this devastating disorder. More briefly considered at the end of the chapter are dementias that are often difficult to distinguish from AD and are now being recognized as sharing certain common pathobiological features with AD.

Alzheimer's Disease

AD strikes individuals of all socioeconomic backgrounds and spares no major cultural subgroup. Clinical symptoms may appear as early as the fourth decade, and the age-specific prevalence increases logarithmically, doubling approximately every 5 years. Individuals who reach the age of 65 have a lifetime risk of 5%–10%, depending on the diagnostic criteria used. The onset of clinical symptoms is insidious (Nixon and Albert 1999). Memory loss is most often the earliest symptom. Onset may be heralded by impaired performance in intellectually demanding tasks at work or a change in personality reflecting a response to these early deficits. Depressive symptoms frequently occur at early disease stages in 30%–50% of cases, but depression tends to be mild and usually remits as the disease progresses. As time goes on, orientation becomes impaired and other features—including language and praxis difficulties, decreased spontaneity, and inflexible patterns of behavior—become obvious to family members and colleagues. Delusions or hallucinations are seen in 30%–40% of individuals with AD; hallucinations are more commonly visual than auditory. Tasks that allow the person to live independently—driving, cooking, financial management, and, later, dressing and personal hygiene—eventually require supervision. It has been noted that the loss of specific functional skills during the course of AD occurs in the reverse order from which these skills are acquired during normal development (Reisberg et al. 1998).

By the time the clinical diagnosis of AD can be made by DSM-IV criteria, neuropathology already may be quite extensive in some regions of the brain. The deposition of β amyloid within the brain, a neuropathological hallmark of AD, begins some years before DAT can be diagnosed. Individuals with Down syndrome, a form of mental retardation associated with triplication of the short arm of chromosome 21, invariably develop AD (according to neuropathological criteria) as much as a decade before clinical dementia can be detected. Now that potential pharmacological therapies for AD are on the horizon, identifying the earliest stage at which structural changes and cognitive deficits in DAT can be distinguished from those of normal aging has become extremely important. Certain neuropsychological indicators are proving potentially useful. Poor performance on measures of delayed recall, and in some cases, measures of verbal fluency have been effective in identifying individuals who later developed DAT. Moreover, individuals at increased risk for AD on the basis of their inheritance of the apolipoprotein E (Apo E) ε4 allele have a particularly high rate of conversion to DAT within several years if they also exhibit impaired performance on visual memory and learning retention (Petersen et al. 1995). In longitudinal studies, hippocampal atrophy in subjects with mild cognitive impairment was a highly significant risk factor for subsequent decline to dementia within 4 years (de Leon et al. 1993).

Neural Circuitry in Alzheimer's Disease

Although forms of dementia arising late in life had been identified by Kraepelin and his colleagues in the 1800s, it was not until 1907 that Alois Alzheimer identified a presenile form of dementia. This dementia exhibited a unique neuropathology in which intraneuronal fibrous structures—the neurofibrillary tangles (NFT)—and additional extracellular plaque-like lesions—termed *senile* or *neuritic plaques*—coexisted in the same brain regions (Figure 8–1).

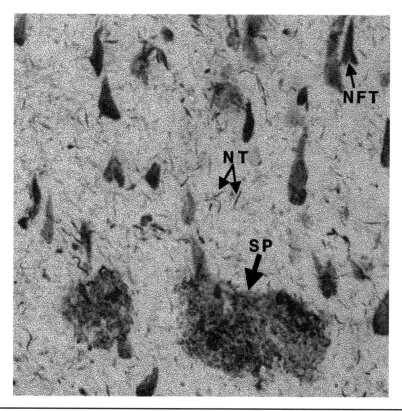

Figure 8–1. *Classic neuropathological lesions in Alzheimer's disease. This section from prefrontal cortex is from a patient with Alzheimer's disease and is immunostained for tau protein* **(black)** *and the Aβ polypeptide* **(brown)**, *illustrating the two defining lesions of the disease. Neurofibrillary tangles (NFT) in neuronal perikarya and neuropil threads (NT) in the processes of affected neurons are composed mainly of tau-containing paired helical filaments. Flame-shaped "ghost" tangles persist long after the neuron in which they developed has died. The extracellular space contains deposits of β-amyloid, a fibrillary form of Aβ. When associated with dystrophic or degenerating neurites containing abnormal tau forms, these lesions are termed neuritic plaques or senile plaques (SP). In sufficient numbers, these plaques in the brain are pathognomonic of Alzheimer's disease.*

The neurofibrillary tangles first identified by Alzheimer are now known to be skeins of twisted abnormal filaments whose presence in neurons reflects a global disorganization of the neuronal cytoskeleton (Goedert 1993). The abnormal filaments, which assume a paired helical structure, are composed of the microtubule-associated tau protein and are present in a hyperphosphorylated state. The paired helical filaments coexist in tangles with fragments of various cytoskeletal proteins. When found in neurites (axons and dendrites), these filaments are referred to as *neuropil threads* and are a defining feature of the dystrophic neurites abundant within neuritic plaques. The appearance of neuropil threads earlier than NFT reflects the slow progression of cellular compromise from the synapse endings toward the neuronal perikaryon over several or more years. This centrifugal progression of degeneration implies that synaptic function becomes impaired well before the neuron is lost.

A second neuropathological hallmark of AD is the presence of *neuritic plaques,* which are complex spherical lesions of varying sizes, usually many times larger than a single neuron. These typically contain an extracellular core of β amyloid surrounded by dystrophic dendrites and axons as well as phagocytic cells of various types (Mann et al. 1998). Fibrils within these plaques are principally composed of β-amyloid peptide (Aβ), a 40- to 43-amino-acid peptide derived from the normal processing of a larger ubiquitous membrane glycoprotein, the β-amyloid precursor protein (βAPP) (Checler 1995). In addition to containing abundant Aβ, neuritic plaques are composed of a host of other proteins and protein fragments derived from degenerating cells or liberated from reactive astrocytes and phagocytic cells. Diffuse plaques containing nonfibrillar deposits of Aβ may appear several years before the neuritic plaques. The relationship of these diffuse Aβ deposits to the development of neuritic plaques is still not understood. Diffuse plaques may be widespread throughout the brains of elderly individuals with no measurable cognitive impairment. By contrast, neuritic plaques are primarily confined to the neocortex, hippocampus, and amygdala (Mann 1997).

The diagnosis of AD is based on histopathological rather than clinical criteria. According to one set of criteria, a definite diagnosis of AD can be made only when neuritic plaques reach a requisite number, adjusted for age, in the most affected regions of the neocortex (Mirra et al. 1991). More stringent research criteria require quantification of both neuritic plaques and neurofibrillary tangles. Controversy has existed over how well plaque density correlates with the cognitive alterations in AD. The appearance and progression of NFT follow a consistent cytoarchitechtonic pattern that parallels the severity of clinical dementia and neuronal cell loss more closely than does the evolution of senile plaques (Arnold et al. 1991; Braak and Braak 1991; Gomez-Isla et al. 1996). The trans-entorhinal region, particularly layers II and IV of the entorhinal cortex, usually shows the first lesions in AD. By the time the mildest stage of cognitive impairment is detectable, the entorhinal cortex may have one-third fewer neurons than normal. Extrapolations from the rate of subsequent fallout of this cell population suggest that neuronal loss may begin as much as 7–10 years before symptoms are detectable.

The highly predictable development of neurofibrillary degeneration in the entorhinal cortex and its progressive extension into the hippocampus, neocortex, and later into various subcortical structures was the basis for a pathology staging system developed by Braak and Braak (1991, 1997). This system uses cross-sectional data on NFT distribution to distinguish six stages of disease evolution. According to this scheme, disease begins in stage 1 with the involvement of only a few trans-entorhinal projection cells, and progresses in stage 2 to involve many entorhinal neurons, particularly those in layer II. Because the superficial cell layers of the entorhinal and perirhinal cortex give rise to the perforant pathway, the final common projection for essentially all cortically derived information to the hippocampus, this destruction essentially removes afferent connections to the hippocampus (Gomez-Isla et al. 1996). At this stage, however, obvious impairment of intellectual capacities is still minimal (Braak and Braak 1997). In stages 3 and 4, neurofibrillary degeneration remains restricted to limbic regions but now begins to invade the hippocampal formation. Degeneration of neurons in the CA1 subfield of the hippocampus in AD is of particular interest, because this hippocampal region experiences no cell loss in normal aging. The two principal targets of the CA1/subicular projection are the accessory nucleus of the amygdala and layer IV of the entorhinal cortex, which provide the principal output from the hippocampus to cortical and subcortical regions. Thus, the progression of changes to these targets in stage 4 gradually isolates the hippocampus from other brain structures. Although many patients in stages 3 and 4 will not yet meet neuropathological criteria for AD, these anatomic changes are associated with impaired cognitive functioning and subtle changes in personality in some individuals. By stage 5, cognitive deficits have become broader, and the clinical diagnosis of DAT can usually be confirmed by neuropathological criteria. At this point, NFT have increasingly appeared in projection neurons within layers II, III, and V of the higher-order association cortices (Arnold et al. 1991), beginning with the temporal lobe, which is more severely affected than the parietal and frontal association cortices. Large cortical projection neurons in layers III and V exhibit the most prominent cytoskeletal alterations, and these cells may be lost to a greater degree than smaller neurons. This pattern of cell loss reflects the special vulnerability of feedforward and feedback circuitry linking the hemispheres with each other and with the cortex of the limbic lobe and subcortical structures. The basis for this selective vulnerability is poorly understood but may be related, in part, to features of the cytoskeleton in distinct cortical projection neurons (Morrison et al. 1998).

Although the cerebral cortex is the primary target in AD, degeneration of subcortical structures may also contribute to memory impairment and behavioral disturbances (Damasio 1984; Mann 1997). The nucleus basalis of Meynert provides the major cholinergic input to the cortex and is important for memory, but the variability and timing of cholinergic changes suggest that they are not a key factor in early cognitive impairment (Haroutunian et al. 1998). The amygdala receives prominent projections from cortical areas and subcortical areas; degeneration therein is particularly relevant to disease-related impairments in motivated and emotional behavior. Extensive cell loss in the noradrenergic locus coeruleus, which richly innervates the cortex, has been associated with depressive symptoms. Changes in the serotonergic raphe nuclei and involvement of hypothalamic nuclei, including the suprachiasmatic nucleus, may explain the impairments of sleep and circadian rhythm commonly observed in AD. Although dopaminergic neurons of the ventral tegmentum are severely depleted, cell loss is only moderate in the substantia nigra, as reflected by the absence of Lewy body pathology and associated extrapyramidal symptoms. The well-documented reduction in levels of various neurotransmitters and their receptors (Young and Penney 1994) is almost certainly a secondary consequence of the loss or functional deafferentation of these subcortical projection neurons.

Signaling Pathways in Alzheimer's Disease

Relevant Genes and Proteins

Recent genetic advances have shown AD to be the common pathological outcome of a family of diseases with different primary etiologies (Cruts and Van Broeckhoven 1998). Gene mutations on at least three different chromosomes account for the familial forms of AD. Roughly one-third of patients with AD have a familial predisposition, with at least one other affected first-degree relative. In families with early-onset AD (arising before the age of 65), which accounts for 2%–10% of all AD cases, the transmission pattern is consistent with an autosomal dominant disorder with age-dependent penetrance. In families with late-onset AD and in the 60%–75% of AD cases that are considered "sporadic," emergence of disease is influenced by various environmental factors as well as by multiple genes with either neuroprotective or disease-facilitatory effects. To date, early-onset familial AD has been linked to mutations of three different genes: the APP gene, and the presenilin 1 (PS1) and presenilin 2 (PS2) genes. Together, these mutations account for

30%–50% of cases of autosomal dominant early-onset AD. In addition, the ε4 allele of the Apo E gene has been identified as a genetic risk factor for both early- and late-onset AD.

The identification of mutations in the APP gene as a rare cause of early-onset AD came on the heels of the discovery that the Aβ peptide is generated by proteolytic cleavage of the APP molecule. Additionally, other findings have established that the APP gene is located within the region of chromosome 21 that is triplicated in Down syndrome, a genetic abnormality associated with high risk for AD. Discovery of the first APP mutation found to cause early-onset AD, the val 717ile "London" mutation, was followed by identification of six additional AD-related APP mutations in or around the Aβ sequence in early-onset-AD families (Hardy 1997).

APP is a housekeeping gene that encodes a single membrane-spanning protein with a large extracellular domain and a small cytoplasmic tail. APP appears to be a member of a larger family of similar proteins that share some of its biological activities but lack the Aβ sequence. Its ubiquitous tissue expression and relatively conserved structure suggest important biological roles, although the major functions of APP and of its major secreted derivative, sAPP-α, remain unclear. Alternative splicing of the APP gene yields three transcripts that encode molecules containing 695, 751, or 770 amino acids. APP_{770} and $βAPP_{751}$ contain a 56-amino-acid domain resembling a serine protease inhibitor. As discussed in the next section, hypotheses about how APP acts as an etiological factor in AD focus on either loss of one of APP's still-unknown functions or a neurotoxic effect of processed derivatives of APP (i.e., gain of negative function).

Missense mutations of the PS1 and PS2 genes result in an aggressive, early-onset form of AD, usually beginning between the ages of 40 and 60 years. PS1, located on chromosome 14, contains 13 exons encoding a 467-amino-acid integral membrane protein with six to eight transmembrane domains (Price et al. 1998). In contrast to APP mutations, the more than 80 different PS1 mutations are scattered over the entire coding region of the gene. Mutations at six different sites have been identified on the PS2 gene, a close homologue of the PS1 gene located on chromosome 1 (Cruts and Van Broeckhoven 1998). PS1 and PS2 proteins are widely distributed among mammalian tissues and are principally located within the endoplasmic reticulum and Golgi complex. In C. elegans, a homologue of presenilin facilitates a signaling pathway that determines cell fate in development. Targeted ablation of the PS1 gene in mice produces an embryonic-lethal phenotype characterized by severely disordered cell division and axioskeletal development as well as selective neurodevelopmental changes in the forebrain. It remains unclear whether the effects of AD-linked PS1 gene mutations reflect a loss of function or a gain of negative function of the mutant presenilin molecule (Price et al. 1998).

A growing number of genes have been shown to influence the risk of developing late-onset AD. Topping the list of factors that increase AD risk is inheritance of the ε4 allele of the gene encoding Apo E, a protein that transports cholesterol and certain phospholipids into cells (Mahley 1988; Roses 1998). Apo E is a constituent of several plasma lipoproteins (very-low-density lipoproteins [VLDL] and high-density lipoproteins [HDL]) and mediates the cellular uptake of lipid complexes through interaction with the Apo B/E (low-density lipoprotein [LDL]) receptor and several related tissue-specific receptors. The virtual absence of other key plasma apolipoproteins such as Apo A1, C1, and B in the brain emphasizes the critical role of Apo E in this tissue. The three Apo E isoforms—ε2, ε3, and ε4—vary by only a single amino acid substitution but are markedly different in their binding affinities for LDL receptors and other proteins. The most common allele, ε3, occurs with a frequency of 75%, while ε2 and ε4 occur with frequencies of 10% and 15%, respectively (Cruts and Van Broeckhoven 1998). Inheritance of a single ε4 allele increases the risk of AD threefold, and homozygosity for ε4 is associated with an eightfold increase in risk (Roses 1998). It appears that the Apo E ε4 allele influences the age at onset—lowering it to the 60s and 70s—rather than the duration and severity of the disease. There is evidence that the ε2 allele confers some protection against the development of late-onset AD and Down syndrome. Unlike inheritance of APP and presenilin mutations, inheritance of one or two Apo E ε4 alleles does not invariably lead to AD.

Efforts continue to identify the genes that account for the remaining half of the familial cases of early-onset AD and/or that influence the risk of developing late-onset disease (Price et al. 1998; Roses 1998). Among the growing list of candidate genes are those related to Apo E function and to the endocytic pathway that mediates Apo E and Aβ uptake and APP metabolism/Aβ generation. These candidate genes include the LRP-1 receptor, α2 macroglobulin, FE65, and the lysosomal protease cathepsin D. Although requiring additional confirmation, these associations illustrate that many genes modulate AD risk and may provide important clues to the pathogenesis of AD.

Pathogenetic Mechanisms

The genetic heterogeneity of AD implies that the disorder can be initiated through distinct cellular cascades, which then converge on the final common pathway(s) responsible for β-amyloidogenesis, neurofibrillary pathology, and ultimately neuronal cell death. Secondary and tertiary responses of the brain to the presence of these neuropathological lesions may further compromise neuronal function, making it difficult to establish cause and effect. Current hypotheses of AD pathogenesis tend to emphasize different aspects of this complex multifactorial process; not surprisingly, these "different" views of disease pathobiology overlap considerably. In this section I discuss three current perspectives of AD pathogenesis that emphasize (respectively) pathophysiological mechanisms of metabolic decline, defective cell repair, and Aβ toxicity in AD.

Metabolic Decline Hypothesis

The "metabolic decline" hypothesis suggests that cellular oxidative stress leading to neurodegeneration is a final common pathway of various early metabolic insults originating from different sources. According to this view, metabolic disturbances are both a cause and a consequence of β-amyloidogenesis. The onslaught on metabolic function begins with effects of normal aging and specific genetic factors. For example, aging-related cerebral hypoperfusion leads to reduced brain glucose and oxygen utilization, which in turn impairs energy production at the mitochondrial level and promotes the production of free radicals (Hoyer 1997). The detection of regional hypometabolism in AD patients with mild cognitive impairment suggests that such hypometabolism not only may result from neurodegeneration but also might precede it. Moreover, cerebral ischemia, coronary artery disease, and some inherited mitochondrial DNA mutations may increase AD risk, in part by creating additional oxidative stress through these same pathways (Markesbery 1997). The resulting oxidative damage to proteins and membranes activates degradative pathways, notably the lysosomal system (Nixon and Cataldo 1995), and in doing so upregulates cathepsins and other proteases, which have been implicated in mechanisms of cell death, Aβ production, and cytoskeletal protein modification (Mathews et al. 2001). Free radicals subsequently impair the function of glucose and glutamate transporters and damage ion-channel adenosine triphosphatases (ATPases) (sodium-calcium pumps), thereby reducing the ability of cells to buffer calcium (Mattson 1997).

Calcium homeostasis is further altered by glutamate and other excitotoxins which stimulate receptor-mediated calcium flux. In familial AD, mutations of presenilin lead to the release of intracellular calcium stores. Elevated cellular calcium activates major signaling cascades, including stress-related protein kinases acting on tau and the cytoskeleton. Calcium-activated neutral protease (calpain) systems, which are highly activated in AD brain, contribute to the breakdown of the cytoskeletal proteins, including tau; alter the activity of the protein kinase C cascade and other signaling pathways; and participate in the mechanisms underlying apoptotic and necrotic cell death (Nixon and Mohan 1999). Ultimately in certain cells, mitochondrial damage leads to the release of cytochrome c, which activates the caspases that mediate apoptosis. Familial AD–linked presenilin and APP mutations increase the vulnerability of cultured neurons to apoptosis, presumably through one or more of the metabolic pathways discussed earlier (Mattson 1998).

Defective Cell Repair Hypothesis

Complementary to the foregoing metabolic decline hypothesis of AD is a "cell repair" version of AD pathogenesis that emphasizes a putative failure by the brain to repair the cumulative neuronal damage arising from normal aging processes, ischemic and environmental insults, and genetic factors. The neurotrophic actions of APP or its mobilization during neuronal injury are most relevant here. Cells normally secrete a proteolytic derivative of APP, designated sAPP, that promotes neuronal growth and increases neuronal survival after certain types of injury (Mattson 1997). APP expression and distribution dramatically increase after neuronal injury, ischemia/oxidative stress, head injury, and exposure to toxins. Cerebrospinal fluid levels of sAPP, however, may be reduced (Hardy 1997). Apo E also figures prominently in the processes of cell repair and regeneration by coordinating the mobilization and redistribution of cholesterol needed for myelin and neuronal membrane synthesis (Mahley 1988). Functional synaptic remodeling in vivo is markedly compromised in mice lacking the Apo E gene (Masliah and Mallory 1995). During regeneration, Apo E expression may increase up to 100-fold. The ε3 allele seems to be more effective as a growth-promoting or repair factor than the ε4 allele, which is linked to increased risk for AD (Buttini et al. 1999). Because Apo E is synthesized in glial cells, neurons depend heavily on receptor-mediated endocytosis to internalize Apo E–cholesterol complexes. Notably, alterations of endocytosis are the earliest known pathological manifestation of AD (Cataldo et al. 2000), and polymorphisms of several genes related to the endocytic pathway are AD susceptibility factors.

Aβ Toxicity Hypothesis

A third hypothesis, referred to as the "Aβ cascade" hypothesis, places the Aβ peptide at the center of AD pathogenesis on the basis of its neurotoxic properties in either soluble or fibrillar form. According to this hypothesis, most AD susceptibility factors either cause Aβ to be over-produced or promote its aggregation into fibrils, which accumulate and are toxic (Hardy 1997; Selkoe 1999). The signaling pathways that regulate the metabolic fate of APP are, therefore, presumed to play a pivotal role in pathogenesis (Price et al. 1998; Selkoe 1999).

After APP is synthesized, a considerable proportion undergoes cleavage between amino acids 16 and 17 of the Aβ peptide sequence (Figure 8–2). This generates a large amino-terminal portion of APP, referred to as sAPP-α, which is secreted into the extracellular space, where it may have trophic, neuroprotective, and cell-adhesive properties (Mattson 1997). sAPP-α secretion is enhanced by electrical depolarization of neurons or by activating protein kinase C through the stimulation of muscarinic receptors or possibly other cell surface receptors (Gandy and Greengard 1994). A substantially smaller portion of total cellular APP is cleaved at the amino terminus of the Aβ sequence by a protease designated β-secretase, which produces fragments of 99 amino acids (C99) that contain the entire Aβ sequence (Vassar et al. 1999). The C99 product is subsequently either completely degraded within lysosomes or cleaved by another protease, designated λ-secretase, to generate Aβ. Normally, about 90% of secreted Aβ peptides are Aβ 40, a largely soluble form of the peptide, whereas around 10% are Aβ 42 and Aβ 43-β species, which are readily aggregated and deposited in amyloid plaques (Lansbury 1997). Although various cellular sites have been proposed for the β- and λ-secretase cleavage events that generate Aβ, the evidence is strongest for the generation of Aβ within recycling endosomes from APP molecules internalized from the cell surface. In sporadic AD, activation of the endocytic pathway and accentuated trafficking of proteases to endosomes are early neuropathological abnormalities that have also been shown to accelerate Aβ production in experimental models (Cataldo et al. 2000; Mathews et al. 2001). Additional Aβ 40 may be generated in secretory (Golgi) compartments of the neuron (Gandy and Greengard 1994), particularly in response to certain APP mutations. In addition, a substantial proportion of Aβ 42 can be generated either within the endoplasmic reticulum (Cook et al. 1997) or at other cellular sites (Mathews et al. 2001).

Aβ deposition within senile plaques involves a balance between forces that enhance Aβ overproduction and aggregation and countervailing forces that promote the uptake and degradation of Aβ from the extracellular space. Although familial AD–linked mutations cause varying degrees of Aβ overproduction (Hardy 1997), they may favor aggregation as well, by increasing the relative production of Aβ 42 or mutant Aβ forms that aggregate more readily. Aβ aggregation is also

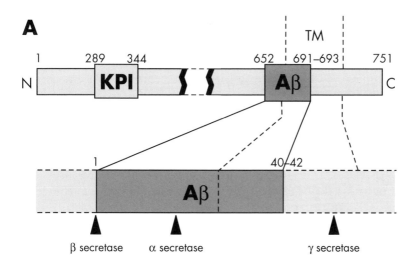

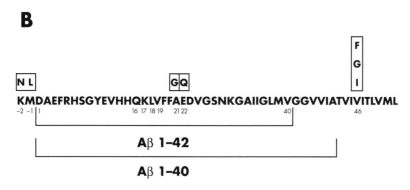

Figure 8–2.   *Structural organization of β-amyloid precursor protein (βAPP) and familial Alzheimer's disease (FAD)–linked βAPP mutations.* **A:** *Upper drawing depicts the organization of βAPP$_{751}$. Kunitz protease inhibitor (KPI) and Aβ sequences are* **boxed.** **Dashed lines** *demarcate the transmembrane domain (TM).* **N** *refers to the amino-terminal residue and* **C** *refers to the carboxyl-terminal residue of the protein. Lower drawing indicates the nomenclature and position of cleavage sites targeted by the indicated secretases.* **B:** *The amino acid sequence of βAPP encompassing Aβ$_{40}$ and Aβ$_{42}$ is presented.* **Boxed** *amino acids correspond to natural mutations observed in the familial forms of Alzheimer's disease: $K^{-2}M^{-1}$/NL, Swedish mutation; E^{22}/Q = HCHWA-D mutation; A^{21}/G = HCHWA-D linked mutation; V^{46}/I, G, or F = other FAD-linked mutations.*

Source.   Adapted from Checler F: "Processing of the Beta-Amyloid Precursor Protein and Its Regulation in Alzheimer's Disease." *Journal of Neurochemistry* 65:1431–1444, 1995. Copyright 1995, Lippincott Williams & Wilkins. Used with permission.

facilitated by additional proteins released by reactive or damaged cells (Mann 1997). In this regard, Apo E is particularly critical to Aβ deposition. Cellular uptake and clearance of Aβ in neural cells involves interactions of an Apo E/Aβ complex with a brain homologue of the LDL receptor, namely the LDL-related receptor protein (LRP). The extent of the influence of Apo E on amyloid deposition is underscored by the observation that Apo E gene ablation abolishes amyloid deposition in transgenic mice that overexpress APP containing a mutation at position 717 that causes AD in some families (Bales et al. 1997). Microglial function also seems to be critical to Aβ removal. In transgenic models of familial AD, Aβ deposition is almost completely prevented when microglia are experimentally activated by immunizing mice with Aβ protein (Schenk et al. 1999).

The fibrillar state of Aβ has been considered to be a crucial factor in Aβ neurotoxicity (Cotman and Pike 1994; Lansbury 1997); however, it is still unclear whether intraneuronal Aβ accumulation or extracellular soluble Aβ forms are relevant to neurotoxicity. Although a sequence of events following Aβ deposition has not been confirmed, it is hypothesized that Aβ accumulation within diffuse plaques eventually leads to local microglial activation, cytokine release, increases in astrocyte numbers, and an inflammatory response involving the classical complement cascade (Selkoe 1999). It has been further proposed that these glial responses and/or any direct neurotoxic effects of Aβ initiate a cascade of biochemical and structural changes in surrounding axons, dendrites, and neuronal cell bodies in AD. Aβ-initiated inflammatory and neurotoxic processes generate excessive free radicals and cause peroxidative injury to proteins and alterations of ionic homeostasis, particularly excessive calcium entry into neurons (Markesbery 1997; Mattson 1997). Aβ is one of various factors that may stimulate the glycogen synthase kinase pathway, which, among other roles, is involved both in the phosphorylation of tau and in still-unclarified aspects of presenilin and APP processing (Imahori et al. 1998). Finally, endocytic uptake of Aβ 42 into cells activates and destabilizes the lysosomal system and promotes cell death.

Thus, although the Aβ cascade hypothesis ultimately reaches the same metabolic endpoints as other hypotheses of pathogenesis, it distinguishes itself by proposing that Aβ accumulation is the germinal event rather than a secondary, albeit important, consequence of the accumulation of metabolic or functional deficits within neurons. To become a comprehensive hypothesis of AD pathogenesis, the Aβ cascade hypothesis must still explain the nature of the initial disturbance(s) that causes Aβ to accumulate in the 85%–90% of AD cases that are not caused by familial AD–linked mutations. Most likely, AD pathogenesis is a multifactorial process in which Aβ is a necessary but not sufficient factor.

Neural Circuitry and Signal Pathways in Other Dementias

Frontotemporal Dementia

Frontotemporal dementia (FTD) is primarily a disorder of presenile onset, developing most commonly between the ages of 45 and 60 (Neary et al. 1998). Within this age range, it accounts for at least 20% of cases of primary progressive dementia, although careful epidemiological studies of FTD remain to be done. Like AD, FTD has an insidious onset; unlike in AD, however, the hippocampus is relatively spared and the earliest symptom is not memory loss. Instead, two types of presentations are seen (Nixon and Albert 1999). The most common presentation, reflecting prominent involvement of frontal and anterior temporal cortices, is a major alteration of personality and social behavior. Lack of conformity to social conventions is often a very early sign. Patients tend to show poor reasoning and judgment, lack foresight, and neglect their self-care responsibilities, including personal hygiene. They may also become either hyperactive (i.e., restless, distractible, disinhibited) or hypoactive (i.e., apathetic, lacking initiative). Changes in eating and drinking patterns as well as stereotyped behavior reminiscent of obsessive-compulsive disorder are common. The alternate presentation of FTD involves early and progressive difficulties with language, beginning typically with word-finding problems and extending to other aspects of language, such as repetition, reading, writing, and comprehension. As these difficulties emerge, the disorder comes to resemble a nonfluent aphasia. In 20% of FTD cases and nearly 50% of FTD cases in which a first-degree relative is affected, mutations of the tau gene on chromosome 17 have been identified (Spillantini et al. 1998). In these families, a parkinsonian syndrome is also prominent, a circumstance that led investigators to name this disease *FTD and parkinsonism linked to chromosome 17* (FTDP-17). Intronic and exonic mutations of tau have been identified that alter either its biophysical properties or the relative proportions of its three splice variants (D'Souza et al. 1999). The nature of tau gene abnormalities in FTDP-17 distinguishes FTDP-17 from AD and other diseases in which NFT are prominent. However, the ability of tau mutations to induce a late-onset progressive neurodegenerative disease underscores that cytoskeletal protein dysfunction can be a primary etiological factor, and this may provide insight into how tau pathology is related to neuronal cell death in AD. The absence of significant Aβ deposits in FTDP-17 also highlights the point that cytoskeletal pathology may be a more inclusive final common pathway of neurodegeneration and dementia than Aβ accumulation.

Dementia With Lewy Bodies

Dementia with Lewy bodies (DLB) is now recognized as the cause of 5%–10% of all dementias, ranking it among the most common types. The intraneuronal inclusions known as Lewy bodies, which are the neuropathological hallmarks of the disease, not only are present in the substantia nigra, as in Parkinson's disease, but also are distributed widely throughout paralimbic and neocortical regions (Gomez-Tortosa et al. 1998). It remains unclear whether DLB is a distinct disease or a variant of AD or Parkinson's disease, because the neuropathological features of AD and Parkinson's disease—senile plaques in AD and nigral degeneration in Parkinson's disease—often coexist with Lewy bodies. Compared with brains from AD patients, brains from DLB patients show much less medial temporal lobe atrophy and greater brain volume reduction. Moreover, DLB brains exhibit little NFT pathology despite having high levels of Aβ. The close association of DLB with Parkinson's disease is underscored by the discovery of mutations in the α-synuclein gene that appear to be responsible for autosomal dominant Parkinson's disease in several kindreds. Recent studies have revealed α-synuclein, a presynaptic protein of unknown function, to be the major filamentous component of Lewy bodies and Lewy neurites in DLB–Parkinson's disease and multiple-system atrophy (Goedert and Spillantini 1998).

The diffuse Lewy body pattern has both diagnostic and potential treatment implications. The clinical presentation of DLB, for example, is often distinctive. DLB patients have been described as having delirium-like fluctuations and cognitive impairment, prominent visual and auditory hallucinations, paranoid ideation, repeated unexplained falls, and transient clouding and/or loss of consciousness (Papka et al. 1998). Consonant with these symptoms, electroencephalographic (EEG) slowing and hypometabolism in the occipital lobe are common and help to distinguish DLB from senile dementia of the Alzheimer's type clinically. Memory loss may resemble that in AD, but the DLB patient displays a greater degree of impairment in attention, verbal fluency, and visuospatial function and is more likely to progress to severe dementia over a period of months. Unlike AD patients, individuals with DLB respond adversely to antipsychotic medications.

Parkinson's Disease

Parkinson's disease is characterized pathologically by a prominent loss of neuromelanin-containing catecholaminergic neurons from the substantia nigra, locus coeruleus, and dorsal motor vagus nucleus. Lewy bodies, the signature filamentous intraneuronal inclusions of Parkinson's disease, are abundant within many surviving neurons in these regions but may also be present diffusely in the brain. Clinical symptoms characteristically include rigidity, bradykinesia, and, more variously, tremor, reflecting the distribution of neuropathology within the extrapyramidal system. Dementia is 6–12 times more common in individuals with Parkinson's disease than in age-matched control populations, affecting up to 35% of Parkinson's disease patients and a higher percentage of those patients who survive to age 85. Parkinson's dementia displays the recent- and retrograde-memory deficits seen in AD but involves greater deficits of verbal memory and greater visuospatial impairments, which can be attributed to disturbed frontal lobe–basal ganglia interconnections. It has been increasingly appreciated that AD and Parkinson's disease exhibit significant epidemiological and clinical overlap and also share certain neuropathological and, possibly, etiopathogenic features (Perl et al. 1998). Although the morphological criteria for AD and Parkinson's disease are distinct, the pathological features of both disorders are commonly seen in the same individual. The presence of Lewy bodies in the substantia nigra is the neuropathological hallmark of Parkinson's disease, although Lewy bodies are seen in various clinical settings and commonly coexist with NFT in the same brain regions. It has been proposed that DLB represents an intermediate variant that would be anticipated if Parkinson's disease and AD were polar extremes of a single degenerative disorder (Perl et al. 1998). The recent discovery of a mutation of the α-synuclein gene causing Parkinson's disease in a large kindred has led to identification of the α-synuclein protein as the major constituent of Lewy bodies in sporadic and familial Parkinson's disease as well as DLB (Goedert and Spillantini 1998). This finding has raised the possibility that altered function or turnover of this protein is a key aspect of pathogenesis in these conditions. It is noteworthy that a fragment of α-synuclein is also a nonamyloid component of senile plaques in AD. As in AD, oxidative stress is considered to be a final common pathway for the multiple etiological factors that lead to the death of nigral neurons. Neurons in the substantia nigra may be particularly vulnerable because of their propensity to generate hydroxyl radicals from peroxide derived from dopamine metabolism.

Vascular Dementia

Cardiovascular disease, whether thrombotic, embolic, or hemorrhagic, may cause regional brain tissue injury that leads to a syndrome of multiple cognitive deficits and focal neurological signs. Most commonly, vascular dementia is caused by vessel occlusion that may give rise to different clinical and pathological pictures, depending on whether large or small vessels are involved. About 15%–25% of late-life dementias in the

United States are attributable to cerebrovascular causes. AD coexists in as many as one-third of vascular dementias, and misdiagnosis of vascular dementia as AD is not uncommon (Tatemichi et al. 1994). Distinguishing these two clinical entities is critically important because many stroke risk factors that predispose an individual to vascular dementia are preventable, and therapeutic approaches to the two dementias are different.

The cognitive and behavioral abnormalities seen in vascular dementia correspond to a frontal-subcortical pattern of impairment. Apathy and inertia predominate. The majority of patients exhibit blunted affect and are withdrawn; they have decreased spontaneity, prolonged latency in responding to queries and commands, and difficulty persevering with tasks that they understand. Patients are laconic and seldom initiate conversation. Patients with vascular dementia report depressed mood, early insomnia, anxiety, and general somatic problems more frequently than do patients with AD. Abnormalities of memory, language, and visuospatial functions are more variable in vascular dementia but are not as prominent as in patients with AD. Although intellectual deterioration is evident in every case, the range is wide. The diagnosis of vascular dementia is made by satisfying the criteria for dementia and demonstrating, in addition, the neurological signs and symptoms or neuroimaging evidence of cerebrovascular disease that is considered etiologically related to the disturbance. In vascular dementia there are often multiple clinical neurological abnormalities. Urinary urgency and incontinence, like gait disturbances, may be early markers of the condition. Parkinsonian deficits such as slowness, decreased associative movement, and rigidity are frequently seen. Typically, there is an acute onset of dysfunction in one or more cognitive or neurological domains, which may be followed by periods of stabilization, or even partial improvement, in functional level, but generally not completely back to baseline. Both the high incidence of AD in patients with vascular dementia and the importance of vascular disease as a risk factor for AD indicate that aspects of the pathophysiology of these two conditions may be additive or synergistic in promoting neurodegeneration. Ischemia, like hypoperfusion (discussed earlier), leads to adenosine triphosphate depletion and subsequent excitotoxicity, as well as altered calcium homeostasis and oxidative stress, each of which would be expected to compound AD-related neurodegeneration.

Psychopharmacology of Alzheimer's Disease

Although success in treating the progressive cognitive deterioration of AD and other dementias has been modest thus far, research in this area is extremely active and encouraging. The strategies being pursued are neurotransmitter replacement, neuroprotective, and regenerative approaches.

A palliative approach aimed at augmenting neurotransmission is necessarily limited, because many neurotransmitter systems are affected in AD and enhancing neurotransmission is not likely to alter the progression of the disease. Nevertheless, many patients have benefited from cholinergic replacement, which so far remains the only treatment approved by the U.S. Food and Drug Administration (FDA) for cognitive disturbances. The rationale for use of cholinomimetic agents to enhance the functioning of surviving cholinergic neurons is well grounded in studies establishing the role of the cholinergic system in memory and learning. This rationale is further supported by studies demonstrating the prominent loss of cholinergic neurons projecting from the basal forebrain to the hippocampus and cerebral cortex in AD. The magnitude of cholinergic deficits, in fact, correlates with the severity of dementia. The greatest therapeutic efficacy among the cholinomimetics has been observed with reversible acetylcholinesterase inhibitors, which enhance the action of acetylcholine released into the synaptic cleft by blocking its degradation. In clinical use, donepezil has largely replaced the first FDA–approved agent, tacrine, because of its more favorable side-effect profile (especially reduced hepatotoxicity) and its longer half-life (about 70 hours). Modest dose-related improvements in cognitive subscales after donepezil administration have been confirmed in several short-term (e.g., 30-week) drug trials with moderately impaired AD patients. The rate of progression of the disease, however, is not altered, nor is improvement sustained after withdrawing the medication. As of this writing, two additional acetylcholinesterase inhibitors—rivastigmine and galantamine—have also received FDA approval.

Cholinergic receptor agonists are also being evaluated as replacement therapies in AD. Of the five subtypes of muscarinic receptors, the M_1 and M_4 receptors are abundant in cortical areas relevant to memory and exhibit unchanged or increased levels in the brains of AD patients. Xanomeline, a partial M_1 and M_4 agonist, has shown efficacy in treating noncognitive symptoms, and trials for cognitive symptoms are under way. The observation that muscarinic receptor stimulation promotes protein kinase C–mediated generation of sAPP-α has raised the possibility that muscarinic receptor agonists might have neuroprotective as well as replacement effects in AD. Nicotine, interacting with nicotinic acetylcholine receptors, may facilitate acetylcholine release and also has modest positive cognitive effects when administered intravenously to nonsmoking AD patients, although these observations require confirmation.

The critical involvement of glutamate receptors in long-term potentiation, synaptic plasticity, and memory and learning, on the one hand, and in excitotoxicity and degenerative phenomena, on the other, suggests their potential importance in dementia. Modulation of one or more glutamate receptor subtypes might have salutary effects on cognitive functioning (receptor agonists) or neuroprotective properties (receptor antagonists) in AD, particularly in view of the marked disruption of glutamatergic pathways in the cortex and hippocampus. So far, however, N-methyl-D-aspartate (NMDA) receptor antagonists, which have well-established protective effects against excitotoxic effects in vitro, have proven to be difficult to administer in humans without serious untoward effects. One exception are recent indications that memantine, a noncompetitive NMDA receptor antagonist, is relatively well tolerated and may have beneficial effects in moderately severe dementia (Winblad and Poritis 1999). Also promising are positive modulators of α-amino-3-hydroxy-5-methyl-4-isoxalone propionic acid (AMPA) receptors (e.g., ampakines) or metabotropic receptors, which have had cognition-enhancing effects in limited clinical evaluations.

A second and potentially more promising therapeutic strategy in AD targets specific cellular events in order to block disease progression. If oxidative stress is a final common metabolic pathway for various etiologically important insults in AD, antioxidants should have therapeutic effects. Some support for this hypothesis was found in a double-blind, placebo-controlled 2-year clinical trial of vitamin E and the monoamine oxidase B (MAO-B) inhibitor selegiline. These antioxidants alone or together slowed (by about 6 months) the rate at which moderately severe AD progressed to loss of basic activities of daily living, the need for nursing home placement, or death. No effects on cognition were seen (Sano et al. 1997). Other therapeutic targets include the processes related to production and deposition of Aβ. The search for inhibitors of β- and λ-secretases has been one attractive approach, although the challenge of blocking a protease that selectively generates Aβ without altering other important metabolic functions of the cell is considerable. Nevertheless, the use of secretase inhibitors remains theoretically appealing. Some progress has also been made in designing strategies to prevent the cerebral deposition of Aβ, which, according to some hypotheses, is a germinal event in AD pathogenesis. In transgenic mice modeling the severe cerebral β-amyloidosis of familial AD, Aβ deposition can be almost completely prevented by ablating the Apo E gene (Bales et al. 1997). Although we may be years from seeing potential clinical applications of this finding, it suggests that modulating the function of Apo E may control the effects of Aβ deposition, including secondary immune and inflammatory responses. Enhancing the ability of microglial cells to clear Aβ is another strategy being developed to neutralize the deleterious secondary consequences of these deposits (Schenk et al. 1999). In transgenic models of AD pathology, immunization of the animal with Aβ has reduced β-amyloid deposition or accelerated its removal from the brain (Janus et al. 2000; Schenk et al. 1999). Considerable effort is now being directed toward evaluating the therapeutic implications of a "β-amyloid vaccine."

The finding of initiation of inflammatory and immune responses at sites of Aβ deposition and degeneration suggests that some aspects of these responses could be injurious rather than entirely helpful to the brain (Popovic et al. 1998). Supporting this view are a substantial number of retrospective studies showing that nonsteroidal antiinflammatory drug (NSAID) use, in arthritis patients, is associated with a decreased prevalence of AD. Some studies, including a small double-blind, placebo-controlled prospective study (Rogers et al. 1993), suggest that NSAID use may delay the onset and slow the progression of AD. Weighed against the side-effect profile of these agents, however, current evidence of NSAID efficacy does not justify their routine use in treating AD patients or individuals at risk for AD.

Retrospective epidemiological studies first revealed that estrogen replacement therapy in postmenopausal women is associated with a lower incidence of AD and that the effect is dose- and duration-dependent (Simpkins et al. 1997). In small clinical trials, estrogens have been shown to improve cognitive performance in women, to moderately slow the rate of cognitive decline in women with AD, and to potentiate the cognitive benefits of tacrine in female AD patients. Large multicenter clinical trials are currently under way. Estrogens have various properties that could explain their possible therapeutic effects in AD (Simpkins et al. 1997). Estrogens enhance cholinergic function by stimulating acetylcholine synthesis and reduce the production of Aβ both in vitro and possibly in mouse models. Estrogens also have significant neuroprotective and neurotrophic properties. In animal models, they attenuate neuronal cell death associated with ischemia and other insults. They also promote neurite outgrowth and enhance hippocampal synapse formation, possibly by means of their ability to increase expression of neurotrophins such as nerve growth factor (NGF) and brain-derived neurotrophic factor (BDNF) and the molecules involved in their signal transduction. Finally, estradiol is a significant antioxidant capable of reducing the toxic effects of oxidized lipoproteins and other sources of oxidative stress on cells. In the context of any hypothesis of AD pathogenesis, therefore, the use of estrogens in treatment would seem to have a strong rationale. Efforts are in progress to develop compounds that preserve the neuroprotective actions of estrogens while eliminating their feminizing effects.

Additional approaches are being pursued to enhance regeneration of injured or lost brain tissue. Progress has been hampered in the use of growth factors as therapeutic by difficulties in delivering these agents across the blood-brain barrier. Because neurotrophins show selectivity for specific neuronal populations and potential for restoring function in experimental lesion paradigms, manipulating neurotrophin signaling pathways, although not necessarily delivering neurotrophins directly, is still considered an attractive avenue for therapy. Another approach, albeit less well advanced, is a strategy to restore brain function by regenerating lost brain tissue or replacing it by neurotransplantation. This approach will likely have the greatest potential benefit for disorders that primarily affect a single neuronal population, such as Parkinson's disease.

Conclusions

The message that seems to be emerging from the intensifying research on a range of dementias is that many different primary etiological factors may trigger one in a limited repertoire of neurodegenerative cascades in a particular vulnerable cell population. Understanding the molecular pathology of one form of dementia may ultimately provide important insights into the pathophysiology and treatment of other dementing disorders. Although serious investigation of the dementias has a relatively short history, research advances have made the prospects for rational therapies exceptionally promising.

References

American Psychiatric Association: Diagnostic and Statistical Manual of Mental Disorders, 4th Edition, Text Revision. Washington, DC, American Psychiatric Association, 2000

Arnold SE, Hyman BT, Flory J, et al: The topographical and neuroanatomical distribution of neurofibrillary tangles and neuritic plaques in the cerebral cortex of patients with Alzheimer's disease. Cereb Cortex 1:103–116, 1991

Bales KR, Verina T, Dodel RC, et al: Lack of apolipoprotein E dramatically reduces amyloid beta-peptide deposition. Nat Genet 17:263–264, 1997

Benson DF: Progressive frontal dysfunction. Dementia 4:149–153, 1993

Braak H, Braak E: Neuropathological staging of Alzheimer-related changes. Acta Neuropathol 82:239–259, 1991

Braak H, Braak E: Aspects of cortical destruction in Alzheimer's disease, in Connections, Cognition, and Alzheimer's Disease. Edited by Hyman BT, Duyckaerts C, Christen Y. Berlin, Springer-Verlag, 1997, pp 1–16

Buttini M, Orth M, Bellosta S, et al: Expression of human apolipoprotein E3 or E4 in the brains of ApoE-/- mice: isoform-specific effects on neurodegeneration. J Neurosci 19:4867–4880, 1999

Cataldo A, Peterhoff CM, Troncoso JC, et al: Endocytic pathway abnormalities precede beta-amyloid deposition in sporadic Alzheimer's disease: differential effects of APOE genotype and presenilin mutations. Am J Pathology 157:277–286, 2000

Checler F: Processing of the beta-amyloid precursor protein and its regulation in Alzheimer's disease. J Neurochem 65:1431–1444, 1995

Cook DG, Forman MS, Sung JC, et al: Alzheimer's A beta(1–42) is generated in the endoplasmic reticulum/intermediate compartment of NT2N cells. Nat Med 3:1021–1023, 1997

Cotman C, Pike C: Beta-amyloid and its contributions to neurodegeneration in Alzheimer disease, in Alzheimer Disease. Edited by Terry RD, Katzman R, Bick KL. New York, Raven, 1994, pp 305–315

Cruts M, Van Broeckhoven C: Molecular genetics of Alzheimer's disease. Ann Med 30:560–565, 1998

Cummings JL (ed): Subcortical Dementia. New York, Oxford University Press, 1990

Damasio AR: The anatomic basis of memory disorders. Semin Neurol 4:223–225, 1984

de Leon MJ, Golomb J, George AE, et al: The radiologic prediction of Alzheimer disease: the atrophic hippocampal formation. Am J Neuroradiol 14:897–906, 1993

D'Souza I, Poorkaj P, Hong M, et al: Missense and silent tau gene mutations cause frontotemporal dementia with parkinsonism–chromosome 17 type, by affecting multiple alternative RNA splicing regulatory elements. Proc Natl Acad Sci U S A 96:5598–5603, 1999

Gandy S, Greengard P: Processing of Alzheimer A beta-amyloid precursor protein: cell biology, regulation, and role in Alzheimer disease. Int Rev Neurobiol 36:29–50, 1994

Goedert M: Tau protein and the neurofibrillary pathology of Alzheimer's disease. Trends Neurosci 16:460–465, 1993

Goedert M, Spillantini MG: Lewy body diseases and multiple system atrophy as alpha-synucleinopathies. Mol Psychiatry 3:462–465, 1998

Gomez-Isla T, Price JL, McKeel DW Jr, et al: Profound loss of layer II entorhinal cortex neurons occurs in very mild Alzheimer's disease. J Neurosci 16:4491–4500, 1996

Gomez-Tortosa E, Ingraham AO, Irizarry MC, et al: Dementia with Lewy bodies. J Am Geriatr Soc 46:1449–1458, 1998

Hardy J: Amyloid, the presenilins and Alzheimer's disease. Trends Neurosci 20: 154–159, 1997

Haroutunian V, Perl DP, Purohit DP, et al: Regional distribution of neuritic plaques in the nondemented elderly and subjects with very mild Alzheimer disease. Arch Neurol 55:1185–1191, 1998

Hoyer S: Models of Alzheimer's disease: cellular and molecular aspects. J Neural Transm 49:11–21, 1997

Imahori K, Hoshi M, Ishiguro K, et al: Possible role of tau protein kinases in pathogenesis of Alzheimer's disease. Neurobiol Aging 19:S93–S98, 1998

Janus C, Pearson J, McLaurin J, et al: A beta peptide immunization reduces behavioural impairment and plaques in a model of Alzheimer's disease. Nature 408:979–982, 2000

Lansbury PT Jr: Structural neurology: are seeds at the root of neuronal degeneration? Neuron 19:1151–1154, 1997

Mahley RW: Apolipoprotein E: cholesterol transport protein with expanding role in cell biology. Science 240:622–630, 1988

Mann DM: Sense and Senility: The Neuropathology of the Aged Human Brain. Austin, TX, RG Landes, 1997

Mann DM, Brown SM, Owen F, et al: Amyloid beta protein (A beta) deposition in dementia with Lewy bodies: predominance of A beta 42(43) and paucity of A beta 40 compared with sporadic Alzheimer's disease. Neuropathol Appl Neurobiol 24:187–194, 1998

Markesbery WR: Oxidative stress hypothesis in Alzheimer's disease. Free Radic Biol Med 23:134–147, 1997

Masliah E, Mallory M: Abnormal synaptic regeneration in apoE-knockout, in Research Advances in Alzheimer's and Related Disorders. Edited by Iqbal K, Mortimer J, Winblad B, et al. New York, Wiley, 1995, pp 405–414

Mathews PM, Guerra CB, Jiang Y, et al: Alzheimer's disease–related overexpression of the cation-dependent mannose 6-phosphate receptor increases Aβ secretion: role for altered lysosomal hydrolase distribution in β-amyloidogenesis. J Biol Chem 2001 Sep 10 [epub ahead of print]

Mattson MP: Cellular actions of beta-amyloid precursor protein and its soluble and fibrillogenic derivatives. Physiol Rev 77:1081–1132, 1997

Mattson MP: Experimental models of Alzheimer's disease. Science and Medicine 5:16–25, 1998

Mirra SS, Heyman A, McKeel D, et al: The Consortium to Establish a Registry for Alzheimer's Disease (CERAD). Part II: Standardization of the neuropathologic assessment of Alzheimer's disease. Neurology 41:479–486, 1991

Morrison BM, Hof PR, Morrison JH: Determinants of neuronal vulnerability in neurodegenerative diseases. Ann Neurol 44 (3 suppl 1):S32–S44, 1998

Neary D, Snowden JS, Gustafson L, et al: Frontotemporal lobar degeneration: a consensus on clinical diagnostic criteria. Neurology 51:1546–1554, 1998

Nixon R, Albert M: Disorders of cognition, in The Harvard Guide to Psychiatry, 3rd Edition. Edited by Nicholi AM. Cambridge, MA, Harvard University Press, 1999, pp 328–361

Nixon RA, Cataldo AM: The endosomal-lysosomal system of neurons: new roles. Trends Neurosci 18:489–496, 1995

Nixon R, Mohan P: Calpains in the pathogenesis of Alzheimer's disease, in CALPAIN: Pharmacology and Toxicology of Calcium-Dependent Protease. Edited by Yuen W. Ann Arbor, MI, Taylor & Francis, 1999, pp 267–291

Papka M, Rubio A, Schiffer RB: A review of Lewy body disease, an emerging concept of cortical dementia. J Neuropsychiatry Clin Neurosci 10:267–279, 1998

Perl DP, Olanow CW, Calne D: Alzheimer's disease and Parkinson's disease: distinct entities or extremes of a spectrum of neurodegeneration? Ann Neurol 44 (3 suppl 1):S19–S31, 1998

Petersen RC, Smith GE, Ivnik RJ, et al: Apolipoprotein E status as a predictor of the development of Alzheimer's disease in memory-impaired individuals. JAMA 273:1274–1278, 1995

Popovic M, Caballero-Bleda M, Puelles L, et al: Importance of immunological and inflammatory processes in the pathogenesis and therapy of Alzheimer's disease. Int J Neurosci 95:203–236, 1998

Price DL, Tanzi RE, Borchelt DR, et al: Alzheimer's disease: genetic studies and transgenic models. Annu Rev Genet 32:461–493, 1998

Reisberg B, Frassen EH, Souren LE, et al: Progression of Alzheimer's disease: variability and consistency: ontogenic models, their applicability and relevance. J Neural Transm Suppl 54:9–20, 1998

Rogers J, Kirby LC, Hempelman SR, et al: Clinical trial of indomethacin in Alzheimer's disease. Neurology 43:1609–1611, 1993

Roses AD: Apolipoprotein E and Alzheimer's disease. The tip of the susceptibility iceberg. Ann N Y Acad Sci 855:738–743, 1998

Sano M, Ernesto C, Thomas RG, et al: A controlled trial of selegiline, alpha-tocopherol, or both as treatment for Alzheimer's disease. The Alzheimer's Disease Cooperative Study. N Engl J Med 336:1216–1222, 1997

Schenk D, Barbour R, Dunn W, et al: Immunization with amyloid-beta attenuates Alzheimer-disease-like pathology in the PDAPP mouse. Nature 400: 173–177, 1999

Selkoe DJ: Translating cell biology into therapeutic advances in Alzheimer's disease. Nature 399 (suppl):A23–A31, 1999

Simpkins JW, Green PS, Gridley KE: Fundamental role for estrogens in cognition and neuroprotection, in Pharmacological Treatment of Alzheimer's Disease. Edited by Decker BA. New York, Wiley-Liss, 1997, pp 503–524

Spillantini MG, Bird TD, Ghetti B: Frontotemporal dementia and Parkinsonism linked to chromosome 17: a new group of tauopathies. Brain Pathol 8:387–402, 1998

Tatemichi T, Sacktor N, Mayeux R: Dementia associated with cerebrovascular disease, other degenerative diseases, and metabolic disorders, in Alzheimer Disease. Edited by Terry RD, Katzman R, Bick KL. New York, Raven, 1994, pp 123–166

Vassar R, Bennett DB, Babu-Kahn S, et al: Beta-secretase cleavage of Alzheimer's amyloid precursor protein by the transmembrane aspartic protease BACE. Science 286:735–741, 1999

Winblad B, Poritis N: Memantine in severe dementia: results of the 9M-Best Study (Benefit and efficacy in severely demented patients during treatment with memantine). Int J Geriatr Psychiatry 14:135–146, 1999

Young A, Penney JJ: Neurotransmitter receptors in Alzheimer disease, in Alzheimer Disease. Edited by Terry RD, Katzman R, Bick KL. New York, Raven, 1994, pp 293–303

Index

*Page numbers printed in **boldface** type refer to tables or figures.*